A Delicate Game

Hana Walker-Brown is a multi-award-winning audio documentary maker, writer, composer and the Creative Director of London-based production company, Broccoli Productions, which was founded in direct response to the lack of opportunities for minority talent both in front of and behind the mic.

Hana is a fearless and passionate advocate of speaking truth to power across all mediums and has covered an exceptional range of true stories, always with human beings at their heart. She is a guest lecturer at Goldsmiths College, University of London and has given talks and masterclasses around the world about her work and creative processes.

Hana has created work for Audible, the BBC, the *Guardian*, *National Geographic*, Spotify and Warner Brothers among many others.

A Delicate Game

Brain Injury, Sport and Sacrifice

Hana Walker-Brown

HODDER*studio*

First published in Great Britain in 2022 by Hodder Studio
An imprint of Hodder & Stoughton
An Hachette UK company

This paperback edition published in 2023

1

A CIP catalogue record for this title is available from the British Library

Paperback ISBN 9781529348088
eBook ISBN 9781529348095

Typeset in Bembo by Manipal Technologies Limited

Printed and bound in Great Britain by Clays Ltd, Elcograf S.p.A.

Hodder & Stoughton policy is to use papers that are natural, renewable and recyclable products and made from wood grown in sustainable forests. The logging and manufacturing processes are expected to conform to the environmental regulations of the country of origin.

Hodder & Stoughton Ltd
Carmelite House
50 Victoria Embankment
London EC4Y 0DZ

www.hodder-studio.com

CONTENTS

To Bonnie, Luca and Theo.
Be Brave.

'The truth is not delicate, and it does not suffer from denial – the truth only dies when true stories are untold.'[1]

Ken Liu, author

A visit to the Midlands, England. Winter 2017

Dawn lights another cigarette and stands in the frame of the back door.

It's our first meeting and five minutes prior to this exchange we were sitting side by side on her sofa, simmering in the silence that her story had left between us. I hadn't intended to talk about it then but Dawn, I quickly realise, does not hold back. An initial chat soon spiralled into her vividly recounting the day her father, former professional footballer Jeff Astle, choked to death, in 2002. She told it with such unflinching courage that it knocked the breath out of me.

'He'd hate this,' she says to herself or to me, holding out the second cigarette balanced between her fingers.

I watch the winter wind pick up the swirl of the smoke. It billows through the crack in the backdoor left ajar, curling around the corners of the kitchen.

Dawn's two golden retrievers begin circling me curiously.

'That one's got a real sixth sense, you know?' Dawn says. 'Knows when a person's anxious or sad and wants to protect them.'

The dog suddenly looks up at me, then rests its head down on my toes.

'Oh bloody 'ell! Not you as well! Christ, what a pair!' She cracks the tension with a laugh, exhaling the smoke like a held breath.

I eyeball the dog, which is still staring at me when Dawn stamps out the cigarette and presses the door closed, rubbing her hands together to warm them as she walks back into the kitchen to click the kettle back on to boil. We chat about everything and nothing as she prepares the tea: the subjects her kids are studying, her former career in the police force, my job and life in London. She can talk, Dawn, and is generous with her detail and humour. I watch her pour the boiling water in the mugs, not missing a beat or a punchline as she goes, only pausing for a moment to let the tea brew.

'Right then, where were we?' she says as she picks up both mugs and leads me back into the living room. We sit side by side on the sofa once more.

She takes me through the rest of the story slowly, methodically and in visceral detail, unfolding the events delicately like fresh linen. She takes her time to walk me through the good, the bad and the unfathomably ugly. And still there is a tremendous gentleness to her tone, to the way she carries me along. She is careful with the details, dates, times and places, deciding early on, for whatever reason, that I am deserving of the full story about her father and what her family has gone through – the whole truth and nothing but.

Her outrage is quiet and considered, while her humour erupts, filling the space and silence, ricocheting off the walls. She segues between comedy and tragedy with ease and there is something about the twang of an accent, the tone and turn of phrase that is 'other-than-London' that I find comforting. Perhaps it's a reminder of home.

'Where are you from then?' she had asked, when I arrived two hours ago.

'A few places – I'm a bit of a mongrel really.' My go-to response to my parents' divorce that feels less complicated than saying a bit Yorkshire, a bit Lincolnshire and a bit London.

'You can't really place my accent, though I'm often betrayed by my northern vowels,' I had told her.

'There's no R in BATH though, is there?!' she had roared. I immediately liked her.

In fact, I'd liked Dawn from the moment I had found a video of her walking out on a meeting with Gordon Taylor, the then chief executive of the Professional Football Association (PFA), after a coroner ruled Jeff Astle's death as industrial disease – the first of its kind – that came as a result of a neurodegenerative disorder caused by the repeated heading of footballs. The meeting took place 15 years after Jeff's death, after the promise of a longitudinal study by the PFA had left the family still fighting for answers.

I liked Dawn then, but I like her even more now, as she flits between fixing cups of tea and taking me through the terror of losing her dad and the almost two-decade-long fight for justice she has become embroiled in. Dawn and her family have been calling for research into football, head injuries and dementia ever since.[2] She's given up her life to hold the sport to account in order to protect other players in the same situation, of which there are now many.

'Football doesn't want anybody to think it can be a killer, but I know it can be because it's on the bottom of my dad's death certificate,' she says. 'And I promised him in the Chapel of Rest that there was no way . . .' she says quietly. 'There was no way I was going to let football get away with it.'

It takes me a long time to find the words.

'They won't get away with it,' I say, with more hope than certainty.

'They won't get away with it,' she repeats quietly.

'Every morning I am reminded of my own vulnerability, my own mortality which in turn inspires me to ask questions; what is life after all? What are we expected to do with this life?'
— Dr Bennet Omalu, neuropathologist

Chapter One

A Controversial Issue

It usually starts with something seemingly insignificant: a curious photograph on a scroll, a conversation on a tube platform, a chance encounter, a text. This story started in 2016 with a text.

Dave Mirra has died! Can't believe it. CTE. Read this x

Had I known at the time that it would end up where it has, sometimes I wonder if I would've opened that message. And yet, I do always open them, the messages. I have an insatiable curiosity about people and the world, and how the two interact. I have spent my career making audio documentaries in an attempt to satisfy my inquiring mind, which has granted me access to the deepest depths of human beings and their lives. I have got on planes as a result of gut feelings that have taken me across continents to some of the most incredible and, frankly, some of the most fucked-up places in the world.

It's a real privilege, sitting down with a stranger to speak until we are no longer strangers. I have sat with their fear, their jöy, their grief, their love and everything in-between. It's a simple exchange. They talk and I listen. Sometimes a problem shared is a problem halved. Sometimes they're looking to lay down their weapons, to let someone else carry the load. Sometimes they're looking for resolution – and sometimes I seek them out, looking for answers myself. I always open the messages that come in, but it's the people I encounter who propel me forward.

This story is no different from that. *A Delicate Game* has spanned years of my life and introduced me to a host of people, from leading scientists to wives and daughters, like Dawn, who have lost loved ones to chronic traumatic encephalopathy (CTE) and have channelled their grief into action, fuelled by a determination to be part of the solution to a problem that is out of control.

While this isn't a story with the happiest ever after, it's one I'm glad I can share here, in the hope that, maybe, it will make a difference.

★★★

So here I am, phone in hand, reading the message, fated seconds away from seeing something that is about to send me down a five-year rabbit hole. I click through to the article, which had been posted on 17 February 2016 on *Outside* online magazine, announcing that, yes, American BMX legend Dave Mirra had died two weeks before.[3] A husband, father and champion rider, Mirra had a ground-breaking career. He won 24 X Games medals in two decades of competition, all but one of them in BMX. He was arguably the best his sport had ever seen.

I had been making a documentary about a BMX club in south-east London at the time. A former DJ renowned in the community, the self-titled Mr CK Flash, had built a track in the park near my house and was training kids from the area to become Olympic athletes. He already had boys on Team GB, including Tre Whyte who would go on to win silver in 2021, and it was crunch time for his next cohort. I was spending a lot of time with the riders on and off mic, having also, very briefly, taken up the sport myself (CK's condition in exchange for handing over his story). I had regaled friends with anecdotes about the track, the kids, CK, and had become accustomed to receiving anything and everything BMX-related. It was a close friend that sent the text. Little did he know where it might end up.

The article recounted how on the morning of 4 February 2016, Mirra had been going about his business, greeting friends at a local bakery and joking about how he was getting too old for the late nights. He had then driven to a friend's house, parked his truck in the driveway and shot himself in the head. On hearing the initial reports, some of his friends had laughed it off as fake news; they even sent messages to Mirra's phone, linking him to the articles to let him in on the joke. For them it was unfathomable. Why would a successful, happy, fulfilled father of two choose suicide with no explanation? No note?

Well, he wouldn't, is the short answer.

A couple of months later, a post-mortem revealed that chronic traumatic encephalopathy, CTE, a degenerative brain disease, had been found in Mirra's brain.

***

Chronic traumatic encephalopathy is a progressive neuro-degenerative syndrome. It is most commonly found among athletes, members of the military and survivors and victims of domestic abuse and is caused by single, episodic or repetitive blunt-force impacts to the head and a consequent transfer of acceleration–deceleration forces to the brain. These can be defined as either concussive or subconcussive blows.

Put simply, concussive blows are the hits to the head that typically cause immediate symptoms: dizziness or blackout. The impact can cause the brain to suddenly shake violently or bounce around or twist inside the skull, creating chemical changes within it and sometimes stretching and damaging brain cells to the point where they no longer work properly.

A subconcussive blow is defined as a head impact that does not result in a clinical concussion, meaning that there are no immediate symptoms. And yet subconcussive blows are believed to have adverse long-term effects in some individuals, particularly if there are repetitive occurrences.

The Cocussion Legacy foundation use the analogy of pitcher's elbow to describe the damage to an athlete's brain from those smaller subconcussive impacts. Pitcher's elbow is a fairly common condition among baseball pitchers caused by repetitive motion and stress at the elbow, resulting in damage to the tendons and ligament of the inner elbow. Every delivery strains the pitcher's elbow, causing micro-injuries to the ligament that builds up over time to weaken, or even compromise, the integrity of the ligament. But this isn't the elbow – this is a brain. The most complex organ in our bodies.

During his career, Mirra had a number of serious crashes including falling 16 feet from a ramp onto his head, crashing so hard he lacerated his liver. On another occasion, he fell 14 feet to the bottom of the ramp, momentarily losing consciousness.

BMX had once been considered illegitimate and unruly – reserved for degenerate kids on the street – but was later embraced by popular culture, although the attitude of the riders has remained the same. They are fearless, willing to take high risks, riding on the edge. The edge itself can be defined as the line between chaos and control, between order and disorder. Between life and death.

A subcultural study of freestyle BMX by the University of Louisville described the sport as 'edgework'. Edgework occurs when the individual voluntarily places themselves in a high-risk situation, or partakes in a high-risk activity, in which the individual could potentially sustain serious, or even life-threatening physical or mental harm if the situation or activity in which the individual participates is not navigated with a high level of skill.[4]

It is the goal of the edgeworker to approach that line or 'edge' as closely as possible without crossing the line or falling off the edge.[5] And it is the proximity to that line that evokes the most adrenaline.

For BMX riders competing, the bigger, impressive, point-scoring tricks require more air; yet, the higher the climb, the harder the fall.

'We ride until we crash,' said Mirra's friend, fellow BMX-rider Mat Hoffman, in an interview with Rolling Stone.

Hoffman, by his own count, has suffered over 100 concussions himself. 'That's just the nature of the sport.'

This wouldn't be the last time I heard those particular words and, as I got further into my investigation, I saw many athletes pushed to their edges – right up to the line for better or worse – and grievous bodily contact consistently celebrated as the ultimate performance of toughness and masculinity.

From the gladiator arena to the boxing ring, athletes have always forfeited their bodies for sport. Often in front of a live audience for money, sponsorship, adrenaline, glory or, ideally, all of the above . . . But *that's just the nature of the sport.*

It was this seeming acceptance and legitimising of violence in sports that initially piqued my interest. I was drawn to the writing of American sociologist Michael Messner who researches, among other things, gender and sports. Messner writes:

> In many of our most popular sports the achievement of goals is predicted on the successful utilization of violence – that is, these are activities in which the human is routinely turned into a weapon to be used against other bodies, resulting in pain, serious injury and even death.[6]

The use of the word 'weapon' was what I found the most fascinating. It implies that someone else is in control, that someone else is using it. I began to explore the relationship between sport, pain and the human body and came, perhaps inevitably, to boxing, a particularly brutal sport in which it is not only legitimate but *necessary* to dominate your opponent by force and violence, channelling aggression to good effect. I disappeared down a rabbit hole into the world of boxing, a sport deeply embedded in our psyche, in our very idea of 'sport'.

Under the Ancient Greeks, boxing was an Olympic sport. They considered it the most potentially harmful of their sports – indeed, a first-century-BC inscription translates as, 'A boxer's victory is gained in blood.'[7] The Romans also loved the sport, which often took place in gladiatorial arenas, with opponents wearing gloves that had spikes sewn into the leather. The loser was the person who died.

With the rise of Christianity, boxing became less popular, although fights no doubt took place. Support resurged in the seventeenth century. In England, pugilist bouts were held in places like London's Royal Theatre. Contestants competed for a purse and fought bare knuckled, but there weren't rules in place. Opponents weren't matched by weight and so bigger, heavier men were at an advantage. It wasn't until the 1740s that regulations were brought in, suggested by the celebrated Jack Broughton, considered by many the 'father of boxing'. He fought for many years under the patronage of the Duke of Cumberland, who, like many aristocrats, had an interest in pugilism. Broughton also invented mufflers, the predecessors of modern boxing gloves, which protected the hands and face. Some people argue that gloves brought more dangers into the game than bare-knuckle fighting, as the contestant was more likely to aim for his opponent's face and head, potentially causing more injury or trauma.

Broughton's rules, introduced, it's believed, because one of his opponents died of fight-related injuries, pretty much served to regulate boxing until the more detailed London Prize Rules were introduced in 1838. During that time, the face of boxing changed, becoming more 'respectable' as the great fighters of the time, such as Daniel Mendoza, Gentleman John Jackson and Tom Cribb, began to get the support of members of the aristocracy for the sport deemed as the epitome of 'manliness' and 'honour'.[8]

The London Prize Rules arguably added to this veneer of respectability for bare-knuckle fighting. It introduced regulations that protected fighters, such as banning kicking, gouging and biting. Fights were also carried out in square roped-off rings and 30-second breaks were introduced after a knockdown, which now signified the end of a round.

So popular was the sport that it soon spread across the Atlantic, taking root in America, although admittedly, the most successful boxers were not homegrown but rather émigrés from England and Ireland. Regardless of where these matches were being fought though, bare-knuckle fighting was still too rough and ready for some aristocrats, associated more with the brawling of the lower classes. Keen to get sponsorship and patronage from the higher echelons of society, in 1867, journalist and sportsman John Graham Chambers came up with the Queensberry Rules, named after the Marquess of the same name. Although scoffed at by some pugilists, the rules were adopted by many, including the wearing of padded gloves and the outlawing of wrestling in matches. Weight divisions were also introduced around this time.

The core organisation that oversaw and progressed sports and sportsmanship was the YMCA (Young Men's Christian Association), established in the 1840s. In both England and America, it offered 'a safe gathering place, opportunities for socialising, Bible-study classes and prayer meetings'.[9] Later there would be greater emphasis placed on physical education as part of their mandate. More recently, their mission statement was updated to 'The Y is the leading non-profit committed to strengthening community by empowering young people, improving the health and well-being of people of all ages and inspiring action in and across communities'. At its inception, it was part of the resurgence of a movement that was known as Muscular Christianity, which I will come onto later, in Chapter Three.

The outreach efforts drew in many, particularly younger men, to box but also to be ministered to, enabling them not only to be part of a team and to work together, but to essentially learn to kneel to authority without question. In church, they would bow to the minister or Jesus in the same way that during matches they would respect and accept that the referee's word was final. As the Edwardian period came to an end, this acceptance of authority became deeply entrenched and boxing even more associated with 'strength, endurance, violence, "sacrifice"'.[10] These same values became particularly important during the two wars that engulfed the world until 1945. It was a game of honour, and in a world rattled by wars, boxing upheld notions of heroism and strength.

In the early twentieth century, it was a particularly brutal sport. The contests were long, with numerous two-minute rounds, and little care was taken to match evenly skilled or evenly weighted boxers. The equipment was poor, with insubstantial boxing gloves offering little protection, which meant that the beatings were severe. Boxers would participate in hundreds of fights in their careers, which sometimes lasted decades. The money a man could make in the ring held an allure, keeping many boxers competing even through injury or when suffering neurological symptoms.

Energy depleted, injuries visible, men would continue to pummel each other until finally one dropped to the floor. If there was no knockout, there was no winner. It was not until 1979 that the New York State Athletic Commissions specified that an assigned physician could step into the ring and stop a bout. There was little thought to the damage done when you're still on your feet, though, through repeated blows to the head.

Detailed accounts from before that time are limited, though we see a glimmer of the severity of brain injury in accounts of a fight that took place in Calgary, Canada, in 1913, between Luther McCarty and Arthur Pelkey – a fight that was supposed to produce a challenger for Jack Johnson's world title. Johnson was the first African American to become heavyweight champion and is considered by many boxing observers to be one of the greatest heavyweights of all time. Pelkey and McCarty were considered 'white hope' fighters ready to take that title off him.

McCarty's match with Pelkey only lasted one minute and 46 seconds. The men circled, they clinched briefly, a few blows were exchanged and then Pelkey struck McCarty with an 'arm blow' – a hit delivered with all available force and muscle power – to the right cheek. McCarty is said to have looked at his trainer and winked (a real showman) before both fighters stepped back and McCarty slumped and fell to the mat. He never regained consciousness and was the first boxer to be killed in a ring in Canada.

A coroner's jury ruled that McCarty had died of a cerebral haemorrhage. It wasn't clear whether the haemorrhage had been a result of a previous injury, which may have included a riding incident where he had hit his head after a fall, or, indeed, of subconcussive trauma sustained from a career in the ring. 'But it was evident that the immediate catalyst to McCarty's death were blows to the head during the fight.'[11] A coroner's jury exonerated Pelkey from any responsibility for McCarty's death, but he was immediately arrested by the North West Mounted Police and formally charged with manslaughter.

And yet, the ruling held that he had not been killed by a blow delivered by Pelkey. It would not be the last time.

In the late 1920s an American man and so-called renowned anti-boxing activist named Manuel Velazquez began to gather data on boxing injuries and deaths after his friend, junior welterweight Pete (Kid Indian) Nebo, was declared mentally incompetent and committed to Florida State Hospital for the rest of his life. He was only 30 and had sustained many beatings during his career. Following Velazquez's death, his data was completed by Joseph R. Svinth. It shows that between 1890 and 2019, some 1,876 boxers died as a direct result of injuries sustained in the ring, an average of more than 14 deaths a year.[12] *Fourteen deaths.* That's deaths, so not counting injuries like those sustained by Nebo. Svinth also noted that all deaths were due to brain injuries. Cardiac conditions, rapid weight loss and so on result in maybe a quarter of current deaths.

Fourteen deaths a year. Fourteen lives destroyed by a moment of incendiary violence in a boxing ring. Why wasn't this taken more seriously? Especially as those deaths were only the ones that came from sudden impact, a cause and effect impossible to deny. But those deaths sat alongside another unfolding disaster, that of CTE. In boxing I would discover the start of the story of CTE, and a template for misdiagnosis and ignorance that would be repeated beyond it.

The foundations of CTE were laid in a condition called punch drunk syndrome, or *dementia pugilistica*, found in boxers. In 1928, a physician and researcher called Harrison Martland published a scientific paper titled 'Punch Drunk'.[13] It described 23 cases of boxers who had started to display neurological symptoms after having experienced repetitive head trauma.

The head trauma was essentially the foundation of their sport; being punched in the face.

Some of the boxers developed symptoms that resembled Parkinson's disease as well as more general types of cognitive deterioration. These symptoms were well known throughout the boxing community. The fans could see it, the promotors could see it; even the fighters themselves could see it. The conditions were often referred to more commonly as boxers being 'cuckoo' or 'slug-nutty'.[14] The symptoms could include confusion, vertigo and a staggering, propulsive gait. The men would eventually deteriorate mentally, often being committed to a psychiatric hospital, as happened with Pete Nebo.[15]

Following his findings, Martland made a plea to neuro-pathologists about the syndrome:

> The [punch drunk] condition can no longer be ignored by the medical profession or the public. It is the duty of our profession to establish the existence or non-existence of punch drunk by preparing accurate statistical data as to its incidence, careful neurologic examinations of fighters thought to be punch drunk, and careful histologic examinations of the brains of those who have died with symptoms simulating the parkinsonian syndrome. The late manifestations of punch drunk will be seen chiefly in the neurologic clinics and the asylums, and such material will practically fall to the neuropathologist connected with such institution.[16]

He also noted that the condition often affects 'fighters of the slugging type, who are usually poor boxers and who take considerable head punishment, seeking only to land a knockout blow. It is also common in second-rate fighters used for training purposes, who may be knocked down several times a day,'[17] drawing a connection back then to the repetitive hits to the head.

Martland's study was not received well by the boxing community and as you can imagine, even then, a phrase like 'punch drunk' was swooped up by the media into a frenzy. By the end of the 1930s, punch drunk syndrome was plastered across the papers, delicious tabloid fodder rather than a serious clinical diagnosis and carrying its own social stigma. In these sensationalised versions, the very real scientific developments weren't fully covered. But did they need to be? Eyewitnesses to the ring could see the effects on the boxers for themselves – the slurring, stumbling, almost regressive nature of the fighters was hard to miss. And since when did the tabloids need facts, anyway?

There were some studies published during the 1930s that explored the 'punch drunk' phenomenon. Dr Harry Parker built on Martland's thesis and presented more evidence of its existence, noting 'punch drunkenness' can present as a 'medley' of symptoms through different symptomatic timecourses.[18] J.A. Millspaugh, a naval lieutenant, published an article in 1937 that presented more examples of cognitive dysfunction in naval boxers who suffered from dementia and disorientation.[19] Millspaugh also introduced new nomenclature to the literature, re-terming 'punch drunk syndrome' as *dementia pugilistica*, which is still used today. Lastly, he analysed the landscape of regulations, rules and precautions taken by boxing committees to ensure the safety of its boxers.

The seeds of discovery had been sown, but as I began to trace their roots, I learnt very quickly that they were given little room to really grow.

A year before Martland's popularisation of the term 'punch drunk syndrome', physicians Michael Osnato and Vincent

Giliberti had published a review of cases of what was known at the time as post-concussion neurosis – a neurological disorder that emerged after a concussion, which established the scientific underpinning of traumatic encephalopathy.[20]

Osnato and Giliberti concluded that concussions could be associated with subsequent neurodegeneration and found that the pathology of the cases studied resembled the effects of encephalitis – an uncommon but serious condition in which the brain becomes inflamed or swollen. They decided to call this disorder 'traumatic encephalitis', which soon became 'traumatic encephalopathy'.

The addition of 'chronic' to 'traumatic encephalopathy' came in 1940 by researchers Bowman and Blau when studying the case of a 28-year-old professional boxer whose career had abruptly ended because he was suffering from numerous neurological symptoms.[21] The boxer's wife reported that her husband had exhibited increasingly childish behaviour and was occasionally depressed. His short-term memory was poor. The patient was described as suffering from paranoia, including times when he felt he was being poisoned, stalked and deceived by those around him. He also had violent episodes and had been arrested for shouting at a stranger. Though he'd wanted to return to his sport, the boxing commissioner refused to allow it on the grounds of the man's poor mental health. It is important to note that the boxer abstained from alcohol, but had experienced many knockouts during his boxing career. The authors initially diagnosed this young boxer with traumatic encephalopathy using Osnato and Giliberti's original terminology; they added the word 'chronic' because his case had not improved over the course of 18 months, leading them to change their diagnosis to reflect this. And so chronic traumatic encephalopathy, or CTE, was born.[22] The condition had a name.

Throughout the twentieth century, there were key discoveries in our understanding of CTE. In the years after Bowman and Blau's research, several studies examining boxers described the 'clinical features of CTE, its relationship to the degree of exposure to fighting',[23] and an array of findings taken from X-rays. But 'each faced setbacks due to issues related to study design, a lack of longitudinal follow-up and the absence of agreed-upon clinical criteria for CTE'.[24] It certainly didn't touch the mainstream in the way that the vaguer term 'punch drunk' had.

Fundamentally, it was and still is hard to quantify the impact of CTE on sufferers: there is no direct measure of the cumulative trauma a person must be exposed to. Researchers Bernick and Banks have refined what they call 'potential surrogates' to this issue,[25] such as the number of fights, fights per year, number of knockouts and the years of fighting.

However, each of these variables may actually have a slightly different influence on the development of CTE. The clinical features of CTE are often progressive, leading to dramatic changes in mood, behaviour and cognition.[26] And yet the first signs would generally appear years or decades after a brain injury has occurred. You couldn't tell when it had happened or how many hits it would take. It's a moot point. Like trying to quantify exactly which cigarette you smoked finally resulted in lung cancer. In some cases, it never will, but with every inhale, a risk is being taken.

There's still so much unknown, so many gaps in the knowledge and inconsistencies. And science cannot be sold or believed when such inconsistencies exist. As I have also discovered, it's often in sports' best interests for there to be such inconsistencies, variables and potential loopholes.

One of the inconsistencies that has caused the most debate is that the disease supposedly presents differently in different sufferers. Some modern researchers have suggested that the disease suffered by boxers is distinct from that found among American football players, for example. This is thought to be centred on a belief that retired American footballers exhibit a predominance of mood and behavioural disturbances, whereas boxers predominantly have motor-related symptoms.

It's true that two of the larger and more influential studies on boxers, including one by Corsellis and colleagues in 1973, focused on motor symptoms. They studied the brains of 15 retired boxers and investigated their lives in retrospect through interviews with the families and found that a characteristic pattern of cerebral change that appeared to be a result of the boxing that triggered many features of the punch drunk syndrome.[27]

Corsellis and colleagues also commented on the mental aspects of the condition: 'Perhaps the more intriguing problems, however, are raised by the psychological components of the syndrome. These have rarely been looked at in the detail accorded to the neurological side.'[28]

Martland, in one of his lesser-known works, 'Intracranial injuries and their sequelae and punch drunk', observes that punch drunk syndrome, as he called it, was not just seen in boxers 'but may be seen in wrestlers, and not uncommonly in footballers'.[29]

There is evidence to suggest that the chronic effects of head trauma in American football, along with the public's awareness of the long-term consequences of that trauma, were being recognised more than a century ago. P.H. Montenigro et al. wrote in the 2015 study 'Chronic traumatic encephalopathy: historical origins and current perspective'[30] that in 1893, a US Naval Academy midshipman and football player, Joseph M. Reeves, after being cautioned by a physician that another blow to his head would cause traumatic insanity, hired an Annapolis shoemaker to fashion the first-ever football helmet.

In the 1930s, cases of punch drunk dementia among football players were noted, including a report of a young football player whose behaviour suggested a 'psychopathic personality' and the 'condition we sometimes find in pugilists . . . pummelled about the head'.[31] This was followed by an editorial in the New York State Journal of Medicine entitled 'Punch-Drunk Boxers and Football Players',[32] which reported that participation in any sport in which multiple head injuries occur, such as in American football, could cause a condition similar to punch drunkenness in which 'attention, concentration, and memory suffer permanently'.[33]

CTE across the early and mid-twentieth century is a story of boxing, but the evidence of its existence in other sports is there, if you look for it. Despite the disparate literature, frequent misdiagnosis and ignorance surrounding the disease, in the years post-1940, the diagnosis of CTE went beyond boxers to encompass athletes from multiple contact sports, including football, American football, hockey, rugby, wrestling, extreme sports, as well as survivors of domestic abuse and military personnel.

All neuropathologically confirmed cases of CTE to date have had one thing in common: a history of repetitive head impacts. These smaller impacts in sport could include a collision of helmets on the American football field, a tackle in rugby, a fist to the face in boxing or the whack of the ball in European football. But isn't that just the nature of the sport?

The Concussion Legacy Foundation (CLF), formerly the Sports Legacy Institute, a Boston-based non-profit organisation, uses the analogy of a car driving down a poorly maintained road. Big potholes might burst a tyre or crack an axle, but smaller potholes do immense harm: they won't pop your tyre right away, but drive over them repeatedly, day after day, and the damage will start to mount. Over time, you'll see the wear and tear and finally the break.

The CLF was founded in June 2007 by Chris Nowinski, a former football player and professional wrestler, and Dr Robert Cantu, a clinical professor of neurology and neurosurgery and founding member and chairman of the Medical Advisory Board at the Concussion Legacy Foundation in Boston. Cantu also consults on numerous NFL (National Football League), NHL (National Hockey League) and NBA (National Basketball Association) teams and serves on the NFL's Head, Neck and Spine Committee and as a senior advisor for the Rugby Research and Injury Prevention Group (RRIPG).

I came to CLF after months of delving into the history of CTE. That investigation often found me coming up short, reaching dead ends or making small moments of progress. That's the nature of the disease itself though – it's never black and white. But then I came across the foundation and in particular Nowinski, who is part of a collective ensuring the discourse and education around CTE and brain injury.

While suffering from extreme post-concussion syndrome following years of injury in the WWE wrestling ring and playing American football, Chris Nowinski learnt that one of the world's leading concussion experts worked just 30 minutes fiom his house. His knowledge of concussion and its impact until that point was minimal, but he knew he was struggling.

> In the sports I played, when you get knocked down you pick yourself up, dust yourself off, and get back out there. I was told if you can walk, you can play. Pain is weakness leaving the body. If it ain't bleedin' it ain't hurt. Suck it up. Take off your shirt, Sally.[34]

He acknowledges that that was the culture he loved and that he would never take a day off just for a headache, but he now questions: 'What had that done to me?'

During their meetings, Chris states that Dr Cantu 'blew his mind' about concussions (although insists no pun is intended). He started with the basics – that a concussion is not actually defined by a physical injury, but by the loss of the brain function that is induced by trauma. That made it much easier for novice Chris to comprehend.

They're an unlikely pairing in person. I watched them deliver a seminar together on concussion before we first spoke. Cantu, with his gentle nature and strawberry-blond hair, arms folded across his chest, tucked into a chair, which seems to envelop him, while Nowinski is broad, almost gladiatorial, his body spilling over the sides of his seat, its back barely containing his body. Cantu speaks in a measured way, Nowinski, too, although his voice is booming, commanding the space. Their respect for each other is easily observed though, each allowing the other to speak first, offering the floor without interruption and directing the questions that are most suited to the other, rather than taking centre stage themselves. Both have played an integral and vital role in raising awareness of

CTE, brain injury and concussion, of advocacy but also of supporting players and their families. They are in the unique position of being able to discuss brain injury within sport on the record, unlike many others who find their research funding tied up with leading sporting bodies. Even so, doing all this hasn't been without its difficulties.

Dr Cantu tells me he thinks its unfortunate that so much research is funded by organisations that have a vested interest in there not being a connection between repetitive head injury and issues later in life. 'Some individuals are connected to tertiary institutions where they are not encouraged to be a part of controversy. You know what I'm trying to say?' he asks me.

I did know. CTE is steeped in controversy, particularly where sporting bodies are concerned, although I wouldn't realise the true extent of that controversy until much later when I would move from reading about those early studies, the first whispers into the disease, to a world populated by big players on both sides. People determined to shape the conversation on a disease that had reached into each and every contact sport.

***

The widely known history of CTE, or the one that broke into the mainstream due to its Hollywood makeover in 2015, is that of the work of Dr Bennet Omalu who famously, or, infamously, depending on who you ask, catapulted the disease into the spotlight after he discovered it in the brain of NFL Pittsburgh Steelers' player Mike Webster.[35] The discovery and his life were later immortalised in the 2015 film *Concussion*, with Will Smith playing Dr Omalu.

'It was an inconvenient truth,' Dr Omalu would tell me with a laugh, 'but the truth is often inconvenient!'

Dr Omalu was alerted after Webster died suddenly and unexpectedly, following years of struggling with cognitive and intellectual impairment, destitution, mood disorders and depression. Dr Omalu suspected that Webster suffered from CTE. He conducted independent and self-financed tissue analyses, which proved he was right. It was the first time a link had been made between CTE and the NFL so publicly and with potentially damning consequences. There would be no apology from the NFL, but rather pushback and a chain of career-defining moments for Dr Omalu that I will come to later.

In 2009, Dr Ann McKee, a neuropathologist and expert in neurodegenerative disease, reported on five NFL players, with symptoms including depression, memory loss, paranoia, aggression, confusion and agitation, who were neuropathologically verified as suffering from CTE at autopsy.[36] C.W. Lindsley wrote in 2017 that 'all five were offensive/defensive linemen or linebackers – positions with significant helmet to helmet contact'.[37] Dr McKee had come into the field of CTE through one of its associated diseases, Alzheimer's.

'It's sort of a Sherlock Holmes type of mystery. You have a patient who comes in with peculiar symptoms, then you want to know the reason why there's a lot we don't know about the brain,' she told me.[38]

'So, for 20 odd years I was very involved in Alzheimer's disease and degeneration and one of the cases that came in was a world champion boxer who was diagnosed with Alzheimer's disease and when I looked at his brain it was fascinating to me because he had a very unusual pattern of tau pathology, the likes of which I'd never seen before.'

Tau protein is predominantly found in brain cells (neurons). Among tau's multiple functions in healthy brain cells, a very important one is stabilisation of the internal microtubules, which help to transport nutrients and other important substances from one part of the nerve cell to another.[39]

When mice are genetically altered to remove the gene that encodes for the tau protein, their brain cells do not function properly and they exhibit motor defects. In humans, tau dysfunction has also been identified as a key player in many neurodegenerative disorders.

In Alzheimer's disease, tau is well known to feature neurofibrillary tangles that are composed of modified tau protein. This means that some other serious brain diseases associated with abnormal tau protein are frontotemporal dementia with Parkinsonism-17, progressive supranuclear palsy and corticobasal degeneration, as well as CTE. All of these forms of dementia are severe and progressive.

In CTE, tau forms clumps that slowly spread throughout the brain, killing the cells. 'CTE initiates focally, deep in the sulci in the cerebral cortex, and spreads slowly, over decades, to eventually spread tau pathology across multiple brain regions.'[40]

It was this uniqueness that propelled McKee to look at more boxers to see if they all had the same pattern of pathology, then coincidentally she was asked to look at the brain of American football players.

'I was very eager to do it because from the beginning of time I was a football fan, having grown up in an American football family with my brothers playing, my dad playing, and so I was very interested in it from several points of view, not just the brain,' she says.

The first couple of cases McKee received involved American football players who were both 45 when they died. The pathology was extraordinary. It looked just like that of the boxer's, only the boxer had died at age 73, almost 30 years older than the football players. This was a shock; football isn't played with the head. What was happening on the pitch that meant the brains of these men were like that of a boxer?

In 2008, the Concussion Legacy Foundation partnered with Boston University and the VA Boston Healthcare System to establish the VA-BU-CLF Brain Bank, of which McKee is the director. It became the first repository in the world dedicated to the study of CTE, housing 70 per cent of global cases. Led by McKee, the research team has revolutionised our understanding of the long-term consequences of repetitive brain trauma and the brain disease CTE.

In 2013, these researchers proposed criteria for the pathological diagnosis of CTE and a methodology for grading the severity of the disease, known as the McKee CTE staging scheme. It has identified four pathological stages of CTE, one being mild and four the most severe.[41]

Stage I can include difficulty thinking and concentrating (cognitive impairment), as well as headaches. In addition to the loss of concentration and attention, Stage II includes depression or mood swings, explosivity and short-term memory loss. This stage could also include executive dysfunction, language difficulties, impulsivity, and the potential for suicide. Those with Stage III CTE frequently develop depression or mood swings, visuospatial difficulties and aggression. Headaches, apathy, impulsivity and the potential for suicide have also been noted.

The most severe stage of CTE, those in Stage IV, suffer from executive dysfunction and memory loss initially and then develop severe memory loss with dementia. Researchers have also found that most of the people studied with Stage IV also developed 'a profound loss of attention and concentration, executive dysfunction, language difficulties, explosivity, aggressive tendencies, paranoia, depression, gait and visuospatial difficulties'.[42]

Less common symptoms include impulsivity and dysarthria – a condition in which the muscles you use for speech are weak, or you have difficulty controlling them, often characterised by slurred or slow speech that can be difficult to understand – and Parkinsonism, which causes a combination of the movement abnormalities seen in Parkinson's disease, including tremors, slow movement, impaired speech or muscle stiffness.

Once it starts, there is no stopping it. There is no cure for CTE.

So many of the possible signs and symptoms of CTE can occur in many other conditions, overlapping with Alzheimer's disease, Parkinson's, traumatic brain injury and various other neurodegenerative disorders. And if CTE doesn't end in suicide, as with Dave Mirra and numerous others, common causes of death for CTE patients include respiratory failure, cardiac disease, overdose and symptoms associated with end-stage dementia, though it doesn't necessarily directly cause these. It makes the disease feel cunning, finding accomplices in those other disorders, with the capacity to embrace all of them as its own symptoms.

It can certainly be suspected, and is, among many athletes now receiving a tentative diagnosis while alive, but a full diagnosis requires evidence of degeneration of brain tissue and deposits of tau in the brain. These can only be seen post-mortem in an autopsy when doctors can slice through brain tissue.

To prove the existence of CTE, doctors, like McKee and her team, systematically search areas of the brain for the unique pattern of tau specific to the disease. The brain's appearance consists of many ridges and indentations. A brain ridge is known as a gyrus and an indentation or depression is a sulcus or fissure. The doctors scrutinise photos of the brain for abnormalities and patterns of atrophy where the sulci and gyri of the brain have become deep or shallow, narrow or wide.

They then slice the brain vertically along what's called the coronal plane, photograph each slice and place portions the size of a postage stamp into microscope slides. The slides are washed in various stains that react to proteins and, in the search for CTE, are checked specifically for the dark brown build-up of tau protein in the brain that can confirm the diagnosis.

According to the CLF, 'the process can take several months to complete, and the analysis is not typically performed as a part of a normal autopsy. In fact, until recently there were relatively few doctors who knew how to diagnose CTE.' And because they weren't trained to diagnose it, they rarely suspected it. From the first discussion in 1928, recorded cases of CTE were rare, conversation within sport was unusual and many, many former athletes were diagnosed with dementia or Parkinson's without further analysis. That's not to say that those diagnoses were incorrect.

The scientific literature on CTE, if you look for it, is vast. It has pulled the attention of the world's leading doctors, pathologists and neuroscientists, people who have found something that they believe, if solved, will save lives – research that they cannot un-see or un-know. It feels to me that whoever you are, once you've become acquainted with CTE in whatever capacity, it's hard to leave it alone, despite the repercussions. But you need to know to look for it.

McKee is the living proof of the all-consuming nature of this story. 'CTE changed me. There's no question. It changed me in a way that I will never be resolved until this disease is resolved. And I'm determined, determined, to do what I can to eradicate it,' McKee sighs. 'It is hard. It's very tiring, because we've been trying to push a ball up a hill or a rock up a hill for decades now and we've made progress, but it seems slow in coming and meanwhile, you know, getting brain after brain in. It's going to require a lot of intellect from very many corners of the earth to really eradicate this disease.'[43]

McKee is diplomatic in acknowledging the pushback she has received for the work she has done; she is calm in the face of widespread denial from the sporting community, which includes some very powerful organisations.

So, it's a hard sell, shall we say.

Ann McKee, Robert Cantu, Chris Nowinski and Bennet Omalu are at the forefront of CTE research and awareness, alongside a host of others that you'll meet in the course of this book. Each plays an integral role in the moments of telling this story, in establishing how CTE intersects with sport and across medicine and the media. Their research and insight cuts through the media perception of CTE, the public conversation as it stands and, crucially, the way sports bodies might want you to understand it.

CTE in the United States has been widely and loudly documented through the media in recent years, in television, books, films and journalism. In 2015, a US district court judge approved a potential billion-dollar settlement that would see thousands of former American football players compensated for concussion-related injuries. But a billion-dollar settlement doesn't make the game safer. It has seeped into the public conscience though, and it was reported in 2020 that concerns about CTE in the US had contributed to a nationwide decline in high-school and youth tackle football participation, as well as local and state-level efforts to ban both activities and a number of NFL and college players walking away from the game.

But for many years the UK seemed quiet. Too quiet.

The public interest has increased around the possible long-term effects of concussions and brain injury sustained during a career in sports, particularly in football since five members of England's 1966 World Cup-winning team have developed dementia. It's led to the deaths of four of them, but in reality, they were only scratching the surface.

Perhaps it's a sign of classic British stoicism in the face of potential adversity that sporting bodies in the UK have failed to address the issue of brain injury enough.[44] And while the FA and PFA did go on to fund research surrounding CTE, by its very nature, CTE is difficult to pinpoint. There are those who would argue that until we know the facts, until we have total clarity, it makes no sense to fearmonger.

But whether it was stoicism, common sense or something more sinister that was stiffening our upper lips, our cousins in America have been, by comparison, screaming about this issue.

If there had been a soundtrack to the rabbit hole I fell down when I started this investigation, it would undoubtedly have been composed by John Carpenter, with notes of tension that alert the body that something is waiting around the corner, minor reminders that if we go a step further, we're in trouble. We know something is coming and yet we still peek through the gaps between our fingers. We can't help ourselves. I felt like that throughout the process of investigating CTE and this work.

Once I knew a little, regardless of how destructive it was, I had to know it all, and once I knew more, I couldn't look away. And it was more than just the material I had or the notes I had made. In his reflections on interviewing, Bengt Bok calls it 'a driving force, an energy ... a will to know'.[45] A will that has its origins inside oneself. I couldn't put it better.

After opening that Mirra text, I spent the following 12 months at least 20 internet tabs deep at all times, amassing as much information as I could from conversations with neuroscientists, pathologists and through my own research. Even so, there still wasn't *that* much information. It existed, that much was clear. It was devastating – clearer still – but I didn't get to the crux of this story, the sense of the real, lived experience, until almost a year after I'd read that Dave Mirra article, through meeting the wife and daughter of a former professional footballer who had died from industrial disease. It's then that this story really began.

★★★

A Visit to the Midlands, England. Early 2018

The first thing Laraine Astle tells me when I walk through her front door is that she's eaten a whole box of Ferrero Rocher since yesterday's shopping run. The confession bursts out of her mouth, the gossip too hot for her tongue.

I rate it, I tell her, which somehow gives her permission to divulge the addition of a Diet Pepsi and a fondant fancy (or maybe two).

'You must've been climbing up the walls!' I laugh.

She nods, shoulders shaking. 'I was! I was like ZOOOOOM!' Her eyes roll back, a pointed finger raised to the roof like a rocket.

'Go steady!' I say affectionately, already enamoured.

Laraine is a talker like Dawn, dropping her guard and immediately putting me at ease, despite the fact that I'm here to ask her the questions. She has the unconditional kindness that grandmothers often possess. I can't take another step without being offered a cake, a slice of freshly made quiche, a tea, perhaps a cold drink? I opt for quiche and we sit with it, plates balancing on our knees, discussing why a lifetime of no alcohol or cigarettes absolutely entitles you to polishing off a box of chocolates and the rest.

'Life would be bloody miserable if, on top of everything else, I couldn't have a chocolate! So, bugger it! I do that. I do rebel,' she whispers with a wink.

Laraine had agreed to see me straight away, following my initial conversation with her daughter Dawn, who I'd contacted via Twitter as soon as I'd seen her walk out on chief executive Gordon Taylor. Dawn's father was the much-admired footballer Jeff Astle, who died in 2002, Laraine his widow.

For over 40 years Jeff Astle was known for his outstanding footballing career at Notts County and West Bromwich Albion, where he played the majority of his career as a centre forward, scoring the winning goal in the 1968 FA Cup Final (one of only seven players in the history of the FA Cup to score in every round). He went on to win five caps for England and was a member of Sir Alf Ramsey's 1970 World Cup Squad. The fans called him 'The King' and he has been described as the greatest football-header the sport has ever seen.

'It was the timing – he knew exactly when to go,' Laraine says, 'and when you see films of him, a fan said it was like watching a salmon rise out of the river!' She tucks her thumb over her index finger, miming the dip and dive of the fish as she speaks. 'It made you wonder how somebody at just over six foot could get up that high. You know, like ballet dancers who suddenly just spring up! Wheeee! You'd think he had ballet shoes on, not football boots! . . . Oh, it was something else!'[46]

Jeff is everywhere in this room. Each of his England caps has a place on the wall, hanging quietly, unassuming, like gentle reminders of a past life, the memories still close enough to touch. Nestled within the biggest frame in the house is Jeff, moments after his winning goal at the FA Cup Final at Wembley Stadium in 1968. He's celebrating in his signature style: both hands in the air, face to the gods, beaming.[47]

Laraine walks me through the life they shared: the first meeting – a disco; the first date – ham salads; the yearly trips to Ibiza; the matches; the goals, so many goals; and then that FA Cup Final at Wembley, including an amusing story involving escaped frozen melon balls from the Players' Wives Dinner.

Once he had retired, Jeff had a stint with Frank Skinner and David Baddiel on the television programme *Fantasy Football*.[48] We laugh together, careful not to spill our cups of tea as Laraine recalls the time that she and Jeff, dressed in matching ball gowns and wigs, were summoned in front of the camera and a live studio audience to sing 'It's Raining Men' to end the show.

'Never a dull moment with Jeff!' Laraine says, rolling her eyes into a smile.

She is generous with her time and tales, and the detail she remembers is astonishing. It's only when we get to the bad bits that I realise why it's been so important for her to keep the good parts fresh and full. If the highs are skyward, then the lows are rock bottom. At 54 years old, Jeff was diagnosed with dementia with onset Alzheimer's.

'It came and it was so vicious, what Jeff had. It didn't come gradually like some did. It was out of control. He plunged into it instantly; there was no time to question, why?'

It had started with forgotten shopping lists and then it was forgotten song lyrics at the end of *Fantasy Football*. It progressed into Jeff having trouble remembering anything, followed by trouble sitting still and then, finally, a trip to the doctor with the devastating diagnosis that would unravel life as Laraine had known it.

'The illness flipped him over. Everything he was, he was now the opposite,' she tells me. 'He had impeccable table manners, Jeff. But now he would just plunge his hand in the butter and plunge his hands in the sugar. Sometimes, I'd come in and find the kitchen floor awash with cornflakes because he'd scoop his hand in the cornflakes, and of course when you push your hand down, they come up like a fountain and there'd be cornflakes over the work surface. He'd have been mortified.'

Laraine recounts other incidents too, such as putting lamb chops to defrost in the kitchen only to find Jeff moments later gnawing at the frozen meat. From then on, anything she needed for evening meals would be wrapped in tea towels and stored on top of the wardrobes in the bedroom. But even once the food was safely in the oven, Jeff would repeatedly open the door, asking if it was ready.

'It was a bloody miracle the Yorkshire puddings ever rose!' Laraine sighs with a laugh, to soften the blow, I think. Though whether it's for me or for her, I'm not quite sure.

There were more dangerous aspects to Jeff's behaviour though. He had unbuckled his seatbelt and opened his door while the car was moving at 40mph down a busy road. He had also taken to grabbing steak knives out of the drawer by their blades.

'Because he didn't know the danger. He'd forgotten,' Laraine explains. 'If I told him he couldn't have them, he'd squeeze them tighter, like a naughty child hangs onto things that they can't have.'

Sometimes the symptoms and stages of CTE creep in slowly, sometimes they come, as Jeff's had, all at once: merciless, like a juggernaut. And still, CTE can never truly be held accountable for its actions until the person in which it dwells is dead.

But at this point the Astles hadn't even heard of CTE. As far as they were concerned, Jeff had dementia with onset Alzheimer's: those were the names they were given. CTE would come much later and not just bring with it years of turmoil for the family but entirely shift the course of their lives.

That Jeff had been diagnosed with such serious conditions at just 54 had felt strange, Laraine reflects, but there hadn't been time to dwell on the finer details. It didn't really matter what its name was anyway; Jeff had been gripped by a monster and Laraine just had to get on with it. She tells me she coped because she had to; the family would rally together to shield his illness from the press, the fans, making up excuses when he didn't show up for match days or appear at the end of *Fantasy Football*. They had a handle on it. It wasn't manageable, but they'd managed. Somehow.

'But then one day I did say to him,' Laraine says, '"Who's that?"' She's pointing to the large, framed photograph of Jeff at the FA Cup Final. '"Who's that?" I said. And that day came, when he had forgotten he was a footballer.'

I look up at the picture.

'I'm just so thankful,' she says softly. 'Thankful that he scored that goal with his foot and not with his head.'

There are parts of the story that Laraine can't say out loud then. That even now, years later, are still too painful to relive. So, that's how I found myself at her daughter Dawn's house, just ten minutes away from Laraine's.

***

The day's light has diminished, the rain now darting against a darkened sky. Another hot tea in hand, I find myself staring up at the photograph of Jeff celebrating his 1968 FA Final Cup goal. *I've seen you like that before*, I think. It is the same photograph that hangs at Laraine's. Jeff is everywhere in this room, too.

'It was here,' Dawn says, now standing beside me to look at the photograph, 'The day he died; it was here.'

Dawn had decided to throw a 'birthday tea' for her father. He and Dawn were born on the same day, so she could easily get away with pretending it was for her.

'Dads don't like no fuss,' she smiles, knowingly.

Laraine and Jeff were late, but this wasn't unusual. It had been four years since Jeff's Alzheimer's diagnosis and each year had been worse than the last. By the time that last party rolled round, Jeff could barely walk.

'He was just a shell. An empty shell,' Dawn says softly. 'He existed. But that was it.'

Once they'd arrived at the house, Jeff was sitting at the table with the rest of the family to eat the spread that Dawn had prepared. She remembers cheese cobs, ham sandwiches and a tray of pickles. I smiled at the mention of cheese cob. 'Where I'm from,' I say, 'it's a bap!'

'Oh, don't you start! Cob, bap, batch, bun – bloody hell!' she exclaims.

Laraine had taken to cutting up Jeff's meals into tiny, tiny pieces like a child's so that he could swallow food without a struggle. He was absolutely fine to begin with, Dawn affirms, silent and subdued but putting the little pieces into his mouth slowly.

'I mean, everything was very slow,' she offers, by way of explanation. In other words, there was no reason to suspect anything was about to go terribly wrong.

But then Jeff started to cough.

'I noticed it very quickly, Dad coughing. I leaned over and thought, *Is he all right?*' But then he started to heave like he was going to be sick. I remember my husband and my mum tried to get him on his feet, and it was winter so, you know, with the heating on it was so warm in the house, and we thought we'd take him out the front door and just give him a bit of fresh air. I remember his legs suddenly buckled, and he was literally like a dead weight. And I think my elder sister's husband tried to hold him up with my husband and they couldn't.'

Her eyes, unblinking, are now fixated on the floor. Her head bowed. Jeff is everywhere in this room.

'Someone shot upstairs to get a pillow and some blankets, and they laid him down and he was – he was, like, coughing and heaving, but his teeth, he'd got his teeth held together and he wouldn't open his mouth. His lips were open but his teeth were gritted together and Mum was screaming at him, "Spit it out, Jeff! Spit it out!"'

She wipes her eyes and looks towards the ceiling, fingers interlaced. It's only then that I realise my hands are clasped together, too.

'There was nothing anybody else could do and I wouldn't say I was particularly religious, but my God, did I pray to God.

Please, God. Let him spit it out. Please, God, don't let him die. His eyes were open; he was looking at you and you were looking at him. "Dad, spit it out," but he couldn't do it.'

Dawn inhales deeply through her nose as if the air around us might will her to carry on. I am still, pins and needles prickly across my palms, having not moved a muscle since she began to tell me about the tea. She stares straight ahead now as if she is watching the next part play out on an invisible screen, conjuring the characters and consequences from behind her eyes.

They're right there, I think. They're always right there. I can see them flicker, memories pooling to the surface of her pupils, shadows shifting across the old portraits of her dear dad.

Another inhale.

'They say because the brain's dying, those signals, they're gone. Like if we want to be sick, you know you heave and you automatically spit it out, but I don't think Dad's brain was sending those types of signals and he choked to death. Asphyxiation on his own sick. The most horrific . . . I mean, horrific don't even cover it to be quite honest with you. All these years later, it does still haunt you.'

'Of course,' I whisper, although I'll never know how it really felt. They're Dawn's memories, not mine, and yet they remain tender to the touch, like a bruise. I don't say anything more, my voice suddenly very small in the room, swallowed up by a silence.

Dawn expels her misgivings with a sigh. 'I wish I had never made that tea to be honest. I blame myself for that.'

She pauses. 'Can we stop there? I need a cigarette.'

She is up and out of the room like a shot; the kettle is refilled, the dogs are let in and she reaches for the Marlboro packet tucked away in the back of a cupboard.

35

'Emergencies only!' she half laughs, holding it up, flicking on the hob to light it.

There is always a moment before you cross the point of no return. Before you have stepped over that metaphorical threshold into someone else's life and story and can no longer walk away. Sometimes it's a physical signal – the breath landing a little lower in the body, a gut feeling, excitement, kind of. Whatever its physical cues, it's a moment that tells you deep in your bones that this is it. There's no turning back.

I feel that in Dawn's kitchen at that moment, suddenly aware of the piles of documents, letters, court papers, photographs and newspaper articles stacked in boxes on the dining table. Each item is a signifier of Dawn's commitment to finding the truth. She couldn't turn back even if she wanted to.

'Oh, those!' Dawn notices. 'Bloody hell, we haven't even got onto those!'

But Jeff Astle's death was only the beginning of the story. Soon after, there was an inquest and ten months later, a consultant neuropathologist would tell the coroner's court that Jeff Astle was suffering from a brain condition that was likely to have been exacerbated by heading footballs.

He found there was considerable evidence of trauma to the brain, similar to that of a boxer, and that it was quite probable that it was heading that had caused it. He himself remembered as a small child how heavy it had been to head a leather football.

'And, of course, once he started to talk about football and Dad's brain looking like the brain of a boxer, the press ... my God, it was like something out of Keystone Cops, because nobody knew. So, of course when they started to mention the word "boxer's brain" and heading footballs ... I can see them now out of the corner of my eye, they have their heads down, writing, and then suddenly their heads would pop up! A unison of heads would pop up, and they scuttled out of the court, trying to switch their mobiles on as they were going. They were quick as anything!'

Dawn animates the memory with her hands, her fingers scurrying across the kitchen counter like little spiders.

'They'd make the call to the papers – "This might be big, this!" And they'd scuttle back in again!'

The family had had their inklings about heading footballs. The balls were heavy, particularly when wet. It wasn't so much the matches themselves – Jeff might have had two or three touches of the ball in a match – as it was the training drills, which were relentless.

The Coroner's Court returned a verdict of death by industrial disease; Jeff Astle's type of dementia was entirely consistent with heading a ball. The occupational exposure had made at least a significant contribution to the disease that caused death.

'Her Majesty's Coroner.' Dawn pauses; there is a shift in her tone now, a seriousness that wasn't there before.

'Her Majesty's Coroner,' she repeats slowly, 'whose job it is to find out how and why somebody has died has basically said that football has killed my dad.'

She places a palm down on the counter as if to steady herself. 'And the press – if they cocked their heads up the first time, it was a double cock the second time – we heard industrial disease, my God! They were straight out the doors again. It was massive.' Dawn shakes her head. 'It was bigger than massive.'

It was the first ruling of its kind. A landmark decision. One that should have had earthquake-like repercussions for the industry. A player was dead, and the cause was his sport.

Brendon Batson was the managing director at West Bromwich Albion at the time and the former deputy chief executive of the Professional Footballer's Association (PFA). He said that the PFA along with the Football Association (FA) had already started a ten-year joint study in 2001 to investigate any possible link between heading footballs and an increased prevalence of neurodegenerative illnesses among ex-professional players. 'We cannot do anything about what has gone on in the past,' he said, 'but maybe we can do something in the future.'[49] I'll come back to this study and what happened later.

At the moment of the ruling one thing was clear, they had an obligation, a duty of care to their players, surely?

Dawn nods. 'We were heartened by that. I mean, I didn't think for one second they wouldn't take it seriously, so you let them get on with it and you try, as hard as it was, to get on with your own lives and leave that side of it to football.

'How wrong were we?'

'If you're hurt, get up. If you fall down, get up. Carry on, kid…
Rugby is like that on steroids.'[50]

— Dylan Hartley, rugby player

Chapter Two

Play On

The photograph of Jeff Astle with his arms outstretched, his
smile wide, running towards the camera in celebration of the
1968 FA Cup goal, has been the defining image of this story
for me. The fallen working-class hero – the King of the Haw-
thorns, as he was fondly known by West Bromwich Albion
fans – tragically cut down by the very sport that made him.

I would come back to Dawn and Laraine after many months
down different routes of CTE, keeping a keen eye on their
story's development, either by email or, more often, watching
it play out on Twitter in 140-character chapters.

It was via Twitter that another image came to sit side by side
with Jeff in my mind, one I had seen Dawn tweet intermittently
on her timeline. A closely cropped photograph of a 14-year-
old boy in his rugby kit, often with the words 'If in doubt, sit
them out' accompanying it. It's this photograph that sparked the
headline 'Death of a school boy' and 'Rugby's Dirty Secret' in
the *Guardian,* written by Andy Bull in December 2013,[51] and

the story of the boy featured in it is central to this book, a gateway into the cataclysmic problem brewing for one of the UK's most beloved and traditional sports. It's an image that has connected so many different strands for me. It speaks to the power, and ultimately the pain, of sport across the ages.

***

That morning of 29 January 2011 had started with an argument, Karen tells me with a laugh. It was 'just an ordinary Saturday morning, filled with bickering over sports socks!'[52]

The socks in question belonged to Karen's two children, Holly and Benjamin, whose school sports matches clashed that day. This wasn't uncommon for the siblings.

'And I said, "Holly, I watched you play football last night so I will run you to school then come back and get your brother. But I'm gonna make the decision to watch Benjamin play rugby today."'

Karen settles into the memory easily, despite this particular Saturday being over a decade ago. I am struck by the rich detail of her recollection, as if each seemingly unremarkable moment from that morning is easy to reach for. She invites me along with her as she retraces every groove. I envisage a warm family home filled with the aliveness of a typical Saturday morning: eggs cooking because all the cereal had been eaten in the week; siblings playfully squabbling over socks; a mother rounding up her children ready for the busy day ahead. A comfortable, familial chaos.

Karen's children, Holly and Benjamin Robinson, were born 18 months apart. They were close and attended the same school, Carrickfergus Grammar in Northern Ireland, where both were avid football fans. Sport was encouraged in their family.

'And dare I say it, not in [Holly's] presence, but [Benjamin] was the better footballer!' Karen says with a laugh. She adores her children, that much is clear, and there's a kindness in her tone, which is somehow elevated by her Northern Irish accent.

'But Benjamin didn't like the crowd or the mentality that went with it,' she continues, 'because it was very much about whose football boots were the more expensive, whose were the best, you know?'

So, Benjamin had moved to play rugby, instead reserving football matches for FIFA on his Xbox. His dad, Peter, had played rugby throughout his life – from school and during his career with the Police. Karen and Peter were separated but amicably and Peter saw his children regularly, often attending their games.

Peter, now a coach himself, also acknowledges that football was Benjamin's first love. 'Oh, [he was a] big Man United fan!' he says. 'Could tell you how much each player cost – he would just hit you with these stats! I just wish his maths would have been as good!' He lets out a laugh.

Rugby was traditionally played in grammar schools like Benjamin's, though Carrickfergus wasn't renowned for the sport, like others in Northern Ireland at that time, but on 29 January 2011, the Saturday that had started with bickering about socks, Benjamin's rugby team were due to play in the Medallion Shield, an annual Rugby Union competition involving schools affiliated to the Irish Rugby Football Union. It was important. Over the years, a selection of players, who went on to win international caps, had taken part in the Medallion Shield final.

Teams entering comprised boys who were under 15 years of age at the start of the school year and born before the end of May. Benjamin was one of the youngest on the team. The match was a big deal; the furthest the school had ever come, something that had seemingly been weighing on Benjamin's mind, since his approach to this match was markedly different to the ones he'd played before. Benjamin was on a conditioning programme to help him bulk up. He would come home with a list of exercises he should be doing, how many miles he should run, which weights he should lift and how often.

The build-up to the match was indeed strange, Karen recalls. She insists that's not in hindsight but rather her mother's intuition with which she knew to worry. Originally, Benjamin's team were due to play on the Tuesday, a match Karen herself wasn't able to make, but it was called off due to the frosty weather.

'And I remember telling him, "Well, that's great 'cause I'll be able to see you play",' she says.

The day before the game, Benjamin had watched *Invictus*, Clint Eastwood's 2009 film about the South Africa rugby team that won the 1995 World Cup for Nelson Mandela's post-Apartheid nation. By the time Friday evening had rolled around, he'd wanted pasta for tea, like all the professional players, but due to Holly's football game running over that evening, Karen felt it was far too late to be cooking that night. The family decided on a takeaway, with Benjamin settling for KFC and an Oreo Krushem Milkshake.

'We sat at the table and Holly wasn't in great form because the match hadn't gone to plan. You can't look at her sideways ... d'you know, that's her in a right strop! She's very passionate! Two totally different kids!' Karen tells me.

Benjamin was the chatterbox of the family usually. He would fill any room with conversation about his day, questions about the world or jokes about his mum's cooking that he often marked out of ten at the table. Karen exaggerates a sigh as she remembers the time she had scored a weak five.

'—and I went, "What, what would make it a ten?" And he goes, "In all seriousness, there's nothing you can actually do to make it a ten, Mum,"' she laughs. 'I said, "Well, we'd best not make that again, eh?" And he goes, "It's probably for the best." A very silly sense of humour – just that awkward 14-year-old stage of being funny and finding his way, you know?'

That night, Benjamin was uncharacteristically quiet though. He was often his chattiest and most mischievous around the dinner table. When he did finally speak it was to announce to the family that he didn't want to let anybody down. Those were his words – 'I don't want to let anybody down' – Karen recalls. All eyes were upon him.

'And I said what do you mean?' Karen starts. 'And he said, "Tomorrow. Tomorrow. I can't let anybody down."' Karen was surprised. 'I said to him, "Benjamin, it's rugby, it's only rugby."'

Benjamin had found rugby tricky at first; he had struggled to understand it. Karen too.

'I said, "I think all you kind of have to do is, like, throw the ball backwards to bring it forwards!"'

When she says that to me now, I agree how absurd it sounds. It's true, the most basic law of the game is that no player is allowed to throw the ball forward to a teammate. In rugby, passes have to be thrown sideways or backwards, while the other ways to move the ball towards the opposition's goal line to score points is by kicking or running with the ball.

Similar to American Football, the object of rugby is to advance the ball into the opponents' end zone. To score, the ball must be physically grounded for a try to be awarded.

Rugby, given its physicality, lends itself to a lot of scrutiny around safety. Naturally, having no protection besides a mouthpiece means players are going to be more prone to cuts, abrasions, lacerations and bleeding. It's certainly not uncommon for players to draw blood during a game.

'Rugby normalises pain and injuries,' said Dylan Hartley, former England Captain in an interview with the *Guardian* in 2020.[53]

I remember seeing his photograph from the 2018 England v Wales Six Nations' match at Twickenham – standing with his hands on his hips, his mouth ajar, streaks of blood running from the side of his head across his eye, ear, cheek and neck, staining his white jersey red. It wasn't for the faint-hearted. But that was in the professional leagues: this was schoolboy rugby, supposedly a world away from the brutality of the big games, not least because the players here were teenage boys, like Benjamin.

Despite Benjamin's confusion with the game in the beginning, by the end of her son's third year, Karen discovered, he had been awarded 'most improved player' at a presentation at school.

'I say "I discovered" because he never told me,' Karen explains. 'It was just a wee small plaque and he had put it in his drawer. So, this is a kid that could take it or leave it. He was starting to understand it a bit more, and he enjoyed it. But if a game was cancelled, well, it was cancelled. It was no big drama.'

Yet, at the dinner table, Benjamin was insistent about his worries about the match.

'I told him that all you can do is your best,' Karen says. 'And if you give your best, you know, whatever happens, happens …

But you know, you have to remember that this is just a game of rugby!'

She suggested an early night for Benjamin, who agreed and made his way up the stairs to bed. It was quiet until a little while later he shouted for Karen, who came out into the hallway. She saw him at the top of the stairs dressed in his rugby kit and the new sweatshirt the team had been given.

'And he said, "Do I look OK?" And I said, "Yes!" And he said, "Do I really look the part?" And I said, "Yes, Benjamin! You look like you always do!"' She says this fondly.

It would take a few more rounds of reassurance before Benjamin would finally slink off to bed. That night he slept in his kit. He didn't want to forget anything in the morning.

'And he certainly didn't want to lose a pair of socks to his sister! Who he knew had a hockey match also, hence the row, the bickering! "You have my socks!" "No, I don't!" "Yes, you do!" "No, I don't, I have mine! You've had yours on since last night!"' Karen re-enacts the siblings' back and forth in mock shouts, but her tone remains kind. For her it was like any other normal Saturday.

On their way up to school that morning, the radio was on. Benjamin had his phone in hand with one headphone in his ear and one out so he could listen to his own music but talk to Karen at the same time. He was chatty as always, the conversation pausing only once when Karen jumped out of the car to get him a Lucozade and a copy of the newspaper. A matchday ritual.

'And we had this thing where he called me Mommy Bear and I called him Baby Bear,' she adds, as if that is the part of the conversation that has stayed with her all these years later. 'And he said, "You know when I turn 15, Mum." I said, "Yes." "I'm going to be playing 18-year-olds." I said, "Right." He said, "Yeah, if I make the first team, I'm only gonna be 15 and they're gonna be 18. I can't be Baby Bear anymore." I said, "Well, you're always gonna be my baby bear." And he said, "Yeah. I know. But I'm gonna have to be buffty bear when I maybe start going to the gym or something."'

The remainder of the journey was spent talking about football, Karen running through the order of the day once again – that she would drop him off, go back and grab a coffee, pick up his stepdad and be back to watch the match. She asked what time kick-off would be, as she often did, knowing full well that Benjamin usually told her 10 or 15 minutes later in case the team weren't doing so well at the start, allowing them time to warm up.

When they arrived at the school, they said their goodbyes, but Benjamin remained in the car, sitting very quietly. He seemed reluctant to get out.

'And I remember thinking, *What is going on in his head?*' Karen sighs. She recalls it turned into a strange morning, a strange morning to end a strange week.

'I think as a mum, you tend to pick up on a lot more than others would. Then that match happened, and it all unfolded after that.'

***

Karen wanted him off at halftime. She remembers when they first arrived, the match had already started, and her first glimpse of the game was Benjamin colliding into another boy. Contact and collisions are part and parcel of rugby.

There are mauls, rucks, tackles – even the words themselves evoke a sense of violence. Rucks and mauls often come about as a result of a tackle.

If the ball and the player is on the ground and players are passing it around with their feet, it's a ruck. If the ball is being held by a standing player, or being passed around a collected pile-up of players, it's a maul.

The purpose of a maul is to allow players to compete for the ball, which is held off the ground. It consists of a ball-carrier and at least one player from each team, bound together and on their feet. Once formed, a maul must move towards a goal line.

After a successful tackle an opponent will stop the ball carrier in his tracks and wrestle him to the ground, effectively ending active play.

Sometimes you might see a player lying on his back clutching the ball close to his chest. A 'ruck' skirmish occurs when a player is on the ground and at least one player from each team is making physical contact above him. Engaging players standing over the ball are joined by their teammates, who come together in the hope that their combined physical strength will surpass that of the opposing team.

Then there is the scrum (short for scrummage), which is a method of restarting play after a stoppage that has been caused by a minor infringement of the laws (for example, a forward pass) or the ball becoming unplayable in a ruck or maul. It involves players packing closely together with their heads down, attempting to gain possession of the ball.

It looks choreographed when you see it, the way the bodies intertwine; limbs tucked around limbs, bones under bone, flesh pressed against flesh, until they become one mound of man – or boy – moving in slow motion until, as if shocked by electricity, the players jolt back into play. The tackles and the scrum are where the majority of injuries occur – fractures, ligamentous tears, dislocated shoulders, spinal injuries and head injuries.

In 2016, Dr Conor O'Brien, a consultant clinical neurophysiologist, reported that there has been a steady and consistent rise in rugby injury rates since the 1950s, when a player could expect to be injured every 31 matches. That doubled to 17 in the early 1990s. In the late 2000s, there was a spike in injuries, when it was reported that a quarter of all elite players required medical or hospital treatment each playing year.[54]

The game is relentless by nature and pain is often normalised. 'If you're hurt, get up. If you fall down, get up. Carry on, kid,' Dylan Hartley had said. 'I teach my kids that. If you fall over, stand up. Brush yourself off. Rugby's like that on steroids.'[55]

The impact and the physicality involved in Benjamin's tackle when she arrived at the match stopped Karen in her tracks. She had never seen him play that hard and aggressively.

'And the impact was such that his upper body kind of whipped back,' she says. I wince.

This wouldn't be the first collision Benjamin would be involved in. There would be a second hit, Karen remembers. Then a third with a boy from the opposing team. That boy cried out in pain and his dad, an off-duty doctor who had been standing on the side of the pitch in a sheepskin coat cheering on his son, beckoned him over to check him out. Dad mode more than doctor mode. On the later collision, Benjamin hit the ground headfirst. He remained on the ground with the referee and the coach, with one of Benjamin's teammates, whose position he was playing in, standing over him, hiding his body from the crowd. He was treated for 90 seconds.

My mind flits to boxing. When a boxer is knocked down, the referee will count over them and the boxer must rise to their feed, unaided, by the count of ten. Ten seconds seems to take an age, any longer and a white towel is thrown in from the sideline. 'Enough,' it says.

If you count out 90 seconds like that, it feels like a lifetime. Benjamin lies there while Karen is pacing up and down the side of the pitch. She knew this wasn't right and she wanted her son off. Benjamin was lifted back onto his feet, he remained on the pitch.

Later the referee would tell the inquest that he thought some of the players were 'prima donnas and drama queens' when it came to injury.

It was Hartley who wrote in his autobiography, *The Hurt*, that 'compassion and coaching are not mutually exclusive, but they don't coexist comfortably'.[56]

Benjamin had been involved in a number of collisions throughout the match, the sheer impact of which Karen had never seen before, and there had been three stoppages in the match so far for Benjamin. Karen had witnessed the coach trace his fingers in front of Benjamin's eyes twice, seemingly to check for concussion. Her son was sent back onto the pitch both times.

Karen remembers Benjamin stood with a big grin on his face. She remembers Holly's friend turning to her and saying, 'Benjamin's not remembering anything.' She catches her son's attention, her eyes locked onto him, when he shouts to her 'I don't feel right!' but he is sucked back into play quickly, there is only a minute left, the pitch rings out with a chorus of shouts to the referee to call the match because Carrikfergus have won, Karen is following the game but it moves away from her quickly to the other end of the pitch. And then the final blow. Benjamin was knocked out before he even hit the ground. Karen didn't need to be told who had gone down. She knew instinctively that Benjamin had been involved in another tackle and was already running across the pitch when his Captain caught up to her.

'It's Benjamin,' he said. 'He's out cold.'

When Karen reached him, Benjamin was on his back, his face was pale and he was fitting. She could see the whites of his eyes.

'He was making a distressing rasping noise and they were still playing. For a few seconds they were still playing,' she tells me. 'And I'm aware of that, because I'm there on my own with him and you know, it could have been three, four seconds, but they definitely hadn't stopped.'

Karen is alone at first trying to keep Benjamin in the recovery position. 'And I keep telling him, "Mum is here, I've got you. Mum is here, Mum is here,"' she says.

It was then that the doctor, the father of the opponent Benjamin had gone in for the tackle with, had come over and said that she needed to take off her coat to keep him warm. 'And it's funny how things stick,' Karen says, 'because I remember looking up at him thinking, *You're wearing a sheepskin coat.*'

The match had now stopped and the coach was calling an ambulance. The doctor in the sheepskin coat was assisting Karen now and Benjamin's stepdad is beckoned over. Benjamin's sister, Holly, was making her way onto the pitch with her friend but Karen had shouted at her not to come any closer.

'And I just remember getting this feeling of it's done, it's over, and there was just an air of it being final. It was done,' she says. The world went quiet, still, it was peaceful somehow. She stands up and goes over to pick up Benjamin's gumshield from the ground. It was almost split in two. Benjamin had a cut lip having taken a kick to the face in the first half and bitten down hard enough to break it. It was calm then, Karen remembers, and in that moment of calm, a woman had passed Karen on the pitch. She didn't know who she was, but she put her hand on Karen's shoulder or perhaps her arm, she can't quite remember, and said, 'I'm really sorry about your son.'

It was then that the calmness of those final moments was replaced by utter panic. Her fear is palpable here now, even to me, a decade later.

That Saturday was not meant to end that way. 'It just wasn't,' she says to herself, quietly now. 'We didn't have great plans, but you know we had Chinese on a Saturday night and we watched *X Factor* or *Britain's Got Talent*. Just some TV, that was the plan.'

Benjamin's dad, Peter Robinson, was at home in Scotland at the time of the match. He had been over to visit and watch Benjamin play two weeks before; he would be there as often as work and family life allowed. He knew the drill for the ones he couldn't make. If Benjamin's team hadn't won, he wouldn't be getting a phone call. He'd have to check up on the result himself. If the team were victorious, he would be the first person Benjamin would call.

'I had two missed calls on my phone,' Peter tells me. 'And then I finally checked in and Benjamin's stepdad said Benjamin's been knocked out. But when you've played the game, you know that these things happen. I suppose my attitude was, well, keep me updated, let me know.'

He wasn't worried; why would he be? That's just the nature of the sport.

But later, it is Karen on the phone,

'And I remember her saying your son's dying. He's dying. And you know it's a very – you're trying to – not believe that,' Peter says, 'but every fibre of your body is telling you differently.'

***

The doctor in the sheepskin coat came in the ambulance with them. He worked on Benjamin with the paramedic to keep him alive. The traffic was against them. It wasn't moving.

Karen says, 'I just remember pleading, you know, please get out of the way.'

The doctor had rung ahead to the hospital to say they had a 14-year-old en-route and that his Glasgow Coma Scale (GCS) was three.

The GCS is a neurological scale that helps gauge the severity of an acute brain injury and aims to give a reliable and objective way of recording the state of a person's consciousness for initial as well as subsequent assessment. It was designed by Teasdale and Jennett in 1974 as a research instrument to study a patient's level of consciousness and to assess comatose patients.[57] It became the method of choice for trauma care practitioners to document neurologic findings over time and predict functional outcome. Before the development of the GCS, there was no standard tool or instrument to assess consciousness levels. This is key: the early detection of complications is critical in avoiding permanent damage; it encourages early intervention. The scale assesses patients according to three aspects of responsiveness: eye opening, motor and verbal responses against the criteria of the scale, and the resulting points give a person's score between three (indicating deep unconsciousness) and, depending on what scale you're using, either 14 or 15 (indicating normal function).

'So, three isn't great,' Karen adds for clarity. 'Zero, it's likely that you're brain dead.'

Karen flits through her telling of the next part, which is full of asides and tangents, the memories harder to muster, blurred somehow through time or grief. Benjamin's pupils were fixed and dilated. She didn't want to leave him. Benjamin was then being taken to a separate room. 'They don't take you to a separate room if it's good news,' she remembers commenting to the nurse. Her desperate need to find her son and not knowing where he had been taken. Finding him in the room opposite. A maze of corridors, consultants and phone calls. Bumping into a nurse she had dealt with in December, having been at the hospital with a domestic abuse victim. The nurse saying, 'This happens all the time; you just have to be patient and be strong for your son.'

Time was stretched and scary – it was all simultaneously happening so fast then slowing right down. She calls it 'an Alice in Wonderland moment', suddenly she felt too big for the building. They remained in limbo, not quite here or there, while they waited. Karen remembers the consultant had asked her what Benjamin had been doing. 'I said we've come straight from the school, he was playing school rugby. I remember them kind of looking at me and I almost felt judged. "You know we came via ambulance,"' I told them. "You know he was playing school rugby."'

She found out later it had shocked the consultants. They told Peter on his arrival at the hospital that they would expect to see traumatic brain injuries like Benjamin's from a car crash, not school sport.

The family were brought up to intensive care and put into an office. The nurse Karen had met before was coming towards them with her head in her hands. She started to shake her head. The consultants would ask again what Benjamin had been doing, proceeding to speak in medical jargon until Karen's husband, Benjamin's stepdad, halted the conversation and asked them directly: 'Just tell us simply, of all the cases that you have dealt with like this, how many have survived?'

The answer was none.

'And I just remember hearing this very guttural wail,' Karen says. 'And it was me. I was making that noise. And it's kind of like looking in on yourself. I was on my hands and knees on the floor.'

Benjamin's brain was so badly swollen with nowhere else to go but down into his spinal column. If he had survived, he would have been left in a vegetative state. Karen tells me that the selfish part of being a mother would say, 'I'll take it, I don't care, I'll take him like that.' But she quickly put that aside to think about Benjamin, what he would want, how he could live in the world after all of that.

The family stayed with him, taking turns to play him music, recalling tales. His cousins arrived, along with his sister. Occasionally the family would be asked to leave so that the consultants could turn Benjamin over or because they needed space for different tests.

Karen recalls moments of being incredibly lucid followed by moments of being very out of control: crying, wailing, fighting and pleading with Peter to get the staff to do something more. She was reluctant to ever leave Benjamin's side but was pulled away as she fought and kicked the walls. She was fighting for her son.

But then there were times when she was focussed, grounded in reality and in doing what needed to be done. It was some time on the Sunday that Karen asked for a minister to come, somehow mustering the strength to organise and arrange the inevitable. They agreed on the Lord's Prayer, biblical phrases. 'God-fearing Benjamin believed in God!' she says with a laugh, but he was also a big fan of music, though there was some convincing to be done. The minister wasn't about to allow anything blasphemous to ring out in the church. Karen assured him that none of Benjamin's favourite songs involved satanic worship but told him to run it past his own son, who was of Benjamin's age, if he was still concerned.

There are moments where she can laugh in the retelling, where the absurdity of the situation somehow takes over the devastation. Where asking a minister's son to clarify that the songs aren't too rude for church feels amusing for a moment until you remember it's for the funeral of a 14-year-old boy.

The school arrived at the hospital on the Monday, two days after the match. The coach and the referee, along with the head girl and two boys from Benjamin's team. The children brought get-well-soon cards for Benjamin, unaware of the severity of the situation and oblivious to the state they would find their friend and teammate in, that he was the youngest person there in intensive care.

'I remember saying to Benjamin, "You know what, son? I think things have got a bit serious here, because the headmaster's here now."' She repeats the conversation verbatim. '"So, Benjamin, this isn't like me asking you to tidy your room and, you know, a week later you get round to doing it!"' She laughs. "'The clock is ticking and they are giving you a certain amount of time to wake up so it's time to wake up now.'"

Two independent consultants arrived to check for brain activity. They injected cold water into Benjamin's ears with a syringe, a test used to determine brainstem death – known as the caloric reflex test. Electrodes are placed around the eyes and connected to a computer. The electrodes are used to measure eye movement during the test.

A small amount of cold water is inserted into the ear canal. This changes the temperature of the inner ear and causes rapid, side-to-side eye movements called nystagmus. The cold water causes the eyes to move away from the direction of the cold water, and then move slowly back.

Warm water is then inserted into the ear. This time, the eyes should move towards the warm water, and then move slowly back. The test is then performed on the other ear. Eye movements are detected by the electrodes and recorded by the computer. Sometimes the person conducting the test visually observes the eye movements.

In comatose patients with cerebral damage, the nystagmus – the eyes' repetitive uncontrolled movements – will be absent as this is controlled by the cerebrum. As a result, using cold water irrigation will result in a deviation of the eyes towards the ear being irrigated. If the eyes don't move in either direction, this suggests the patient's brainstem reflexes are also damaged and carries a very poor prognosis.

The consultants said nothing. There was no response from Benjamin. On 31 January 2011, brainstem testing was carried out at 2.55 p.m. and again at 4.14 p.m. and these confirmed brainstem death.

'He just couldn't do it by himself,' Karen says quietly. After that everything became very procedural very quickly. The family were asked about organ donation, which startled Karen initially.

'I know that I was rude,' she says. 'I said I didn't get a miracle and why should anybody else? No. I probably didn't put it as politely as that even.'

I am taken aback by her honesty, more so when she tells me she was offered diazepam to calm down during the stretch of time at the hospital. It knocks her out for a few hours. When she awakes she is furious with herself to have missed those hours with her son. Though the memory is hazy, she knows she returned to Benjamin's bedside that evening when she was approached again by the donor nurse 'She kept using the word "sudden" and it clicked with me and I said, "Right, OK, so this is a sudden death and you're going to do a post-mortem."'

Karen and Peter had both been in the police force and were accustomed to the procedure. Karen finally agreed to donate certain organs. 'I said, "Right, well, on that basis you can get A, B, C, D and E." And I got the form. They're very generic forms and I kind of went into police mode and I crossed the stuff out they weren't getting and initialled every side.' The operation, extracting the organs, was due to happen the following morning, which meant they were able to spend one extra night with Benjamin who was kept on life support for that reason.

'I suppose we were looking for a miracle,' Peter tells me, 'and then all of a sudden you realise Benjamin's going to be somebody [else's] miracle. We know there [were] five recipients. He went on to save five people's lives. Bittersweet – I must admit.'

Karen told Benjamin what was going to happen, the procedure, the transplants. She promised that she wouldn't leave him, that she would be right there for when he returned. She told him that he needed to do this for Mum. Karen stayed at the hospital for hours and when the medical staff returned later to collect her, she assumed that they were going back to the ward.

'They said, "No, we're going down to another level," and I was not prepared for that. I guess nothing will prepare you, but you've got this scenario in your head that everything is so scenic, and the bed and the lights are there and then things are turned off. But instead, what I got was a room outside the theatre that was really freezing cold, and Benjamin was lying there on a stainless-steel gurney with a sheet over him up to his waist.'

Benjamin had his Manchester United T-shirt on but there were no machines now. There was nothing, except Benjamin and the stainless steel and the cold.

'His hair was soaking and I felt that I had let him down because I told him that's not the way it would be, I would be back at the ward waiting for him, so to be faced with that . . .' Karen trails off, leaving the memory hanging between us in heavy silence. Her train of thought becomes tangled then and I realise how devastatingly hard it is, even now, to try to fathom that this was the outcome of her young son's rugby match.

'I just lost all track of time,' she says quietly after a long pause. 'When I saw him lying there, I didn't realise it was Tuesday evening and, you know, on a Saturday morning your boy is full of life and complaining that there's no cereal left because he's eaten it all during the week and I make him scrambled eggs because he can't go to play rugby on a banana and then. . .' She stops again and with a defeated sigh says, 'I don't know how they got me out of the hospital, I really don't know how.'

Medicated once again, Karen slept in Benjamin's bed that night. She had the coat she had wrapped around him, his patient's property bag with his trainers, rugby boots and the jersey they had cut from him with her. While she slept, Peter, Benjamin's father, had gone by himself to formally identify the body in the morgue. Karen flinches, still furious that she left him to do it alone. For the first time, I can hear her anger rise above the agony; it's only for a second, but it's there. Of course it's there, simmering just below the surface. *I would rage*, I think. *I would rage if I were her.* But she dispels it quickly, calmly, with grace. Such tremendous strength.

'And then we were told he was coming home, and there's that sense of euphoria that your son's coming home. And you're elated! You are beside yourself!' she exclaims. 'Your son is coming home, and again I don't know what I thought. I wasn't thinking very straight . . . But yeah, he's brought home, but he's in a coffin. Your son.'

It is tradition in Ireland to have the deceased washed and dressed and laid in the house ahead of the funeral. Benjamin was wearing the suit he had worn the summer before, the suit he had worn when Karen had married his stepdad and Benjamin had given her away. The tailor-made suit that would be altered for his formal, the suit that Karen tells me made him feel like James Bond.

'So, he's there in his suit and I just remember fixing his hair and then feeling the cold staples in his scalp. I slept with him downstairs.'

When Benjamin returned home, the house became a revolving door of well-wishers, mourners, family and friends. The visitors never stopped. People were coming and coming until the end of Friday, until the family couldn't face it anymore, until someone made the decision around tea-time – Karen can't remember who — that there were to be no more. That the door was to be shut. It had been a week since Benjamin had slept in his rugby kit. The service would take place the following morning. The minister would return to the house first to put the lid on top of the coffin.

'And do you know,' Karen begins, slowly and measuredly now, 'I packed my son off as if he was going away on a trip, his Xbox went in, his phone went in, silly things. A Pot Noodle, a packet of Doritos, money in case he needed it. And when they said, "We're gonna put the lid on," I think I left at that point and all the lights went out in our house. The electrics had gone.'

***

'People used to say that when he came in the room, he made this big smile and he just lit up the room, sort of thing, you know, and, you know. . .' Peter begins. 'He was . . . he would have been a better man than I would have ever been, I can tell you that. The kindest kid.'

At the funeral Karen broke from tradition and carried her own son.

***

When it came to the one-year anniversary of Benjamin's death, the school invited Karen and Peter to a memorial service they had planned. They wanted photographs of him from the family. Their minister had voiced his concerns that it could be traumatic for them to be at the school, surrounded by Benjamin's class and teammates, children who were all a year older, friends Benjamin should have sat among. As Karen and Peter walked into the assembly hall it was laid out the way the church was for Benjamin's funeral.

'I had written a poem,' Karen tells me, 'and I said to Peter, "I really don't think I can do this," and he said, "Well, that's OK, we've told the headmaster that if you're not going to do it, you just give him a nod and he will continue talking."'

Both parents recall listening to the headmaster talk about Benjamin, how great he was, what an excellent player. The vice-principal of the other school Benjamin's team had played that day was there too, with two pupils from the team.

'And at the end, I remember the headmaster winding up his speech and he just said, "Just to remind you that we won the match that day,"' Karen says slowly, and I catch embers of fury on the edge of her words.

I approached the school for comment but at the time of writing this have had no response.

★★★

There would be two inquests surrounding Benjamin's death. Having both been in the police force, Peter and Karen had gone to the inquest expecting to hear the facts. Their son was dead, he had died playing rugby.

A formality that, although devastating, two parents riddled with grief, with their experience in courtrooms, felt they might just be able to get through. But it was never going to be that simple.

'International football is the continuation of war by other means.'
— George Orwell[58]

Chapter Three

The Perfect Storm

'The culture of sport eats protocol for breakfast,' Peter Robinson tells me. 'So, in other words, the red mist of the game, that attitude of win at all costs, you know, play injured and all of that. From an early age, I remember this idea of Just, "Get up and get on with it, stop moaning." That culture still kicks in. I still see it.'[59]

Peter's son, 14-year-old Benjamin Robinson, hadn't wanted to let anybody down when he was playing rugby. The 'most improved player' was aware that he had to carry the team and perhaps even the match on his shoulders. Benjamin had been playing out of position on the day he was injured, instead covering his best friend's, who was out of play with a wrist injury. The team was a player down and only had one substitute that day.

'Benjamin normally would have played 12 on his jersey and he was playing 13 that day. And speaking to his best friend afterwards, you know, and it was a long time afterwards, he said, "That should have been me. That should have been me."' But it shouldn't have been anyone, let alone 14-year-old boys playing school sport.

It was Karen who met Benjamin's best friend at the cemetery, by chance, over a year after the match. Karen came away from the conversation feeling like the outcome of the match had been given greater importance than her son's life.

Since he had been unable to play, the friend had been watching from the sidelines. He had even run onto the pitch himself with a medical bag during one of the stoppages for Benjamin.

He later told the coroner's court he was concerned for his friend, that Benjamin was lying on his back and he assumed he'd been knocked out. 'I did not feel he should have played on,' he said.

Later the referee David Brown would describe Benjamin as the 'stand-out player'.

We are taught as children that when we get knocked down, we pick ourselves up, we dust ourselves off and we get back out there – both in sport and in life – and sometimes that involves making a sacrifice. But how big does that sacrifice have to be? And who makes that decision? In Benjamin's case, that decision, or lack of, proved fatal.

Sports have always arguably served a major role in identity development, but perhaps never more so, in the modern world, than since the evolution of Muscular Christianity in the nineteenth century. A movement that advocated sports and games to instil positive character traits in men, it believed in the physical superiority of males to become 'faithful stewards of God's gifts, to fight in His service, to protect the weak and to conquer nature.'[60] It was characterised by a belief in patriotic duty, discipline, self-sacrifice, teamwork, leadership, manliness and the moral and physical beauty of athleticism and aimed to increase men's commitment to their health and to their faith. Among its supporters were Theodore Roosevelt, who is credited with saving American football after some 20 players died as a result of injuries sustained during matches in 1905.[61]

The author Charles Kingsley, also a keen sportsman, had traced Muscular Christianity's origins to the New Testament in 1 Corinthians 6:19–20, which proclaims our bodies as temples and that you should 'honour God with your bodies'.[62] Kingsley believed that the 'muscle men' mentality of men was written by God himself, making it the most desirable trait, and who was he to argue with the ultimate authority?

It's often documented that the most prevailing worry at the time was that of the 'softening of male morals', which was deemed unhealthy. Sport was considered a good outlet for burning off the energy that might have led men down the immoral path of vice and idleness associated with evils such as masturbation and homosexuality.

Homosexuality was a major concern for public school masters in Britain and so Kingsley's view of a 'manful' Christ, whom he deemed the 'general who is fighting by your side',[63] coupled with his belief that sports and body building were character building, quickly spread throughout the schools and universities of England as an antidote to the perceived problem.

The term, Muscular Christianity, would be popularised in reference to Thomas Hughes's widely read 1857 novel, *Tom Brown's School Days,* set at Rugby School at the time of Thomas Arnold's headmastership. Arnold helped shape Hughes's ideas about Muscular Christianity. In his 1861 sequel, *Tom Brown at Oxford,* Hughes named Chapter 11 'Muscular Christianity' after the concept.[64] Hughes, like Kingsley, was part of the Christian Socialist movement. As a boxing coach, he also introduced an athletics programme at the Working Men's College, an adult education institute founded in London, in 1854, where he later became principal.[65]

Baron Pierre de Coubertin's development of the modern Olympic Games also had strong links with the ideology of Muscular Christianity. After reading a French translation of Thomas Hughes's *Tom Brown's School Days*, and consequently visiting Rugby School, de Coubertin saw the athletic traditions of the English public schools' system as a vehicle for rebuilding the character of France after the Franco-Prussian war and as a model for the rebirth of the ancient Olympics. De Coubertin believed that the importance of the Olympiads was not so much to win, as to take part: 'The important thing in life is not the triumph but the struggle. The essential thing is not to have won but to have fought well.'[66] Such became the core message of the modern Olympic movement. He viewed the sports arena as a laboratory for manliness.

By the late nineteenth century, the movement had reached the United States.

American football's roots can be traced to early versions of rugby and association football, which had their origins in the United Kingdom in the mid-nineteenth century, although there were several major divergences from the sports it had stemmed from. The rule changes were instituted by Walter Camp, a Yale University and Hopkins School graduate, considered to be the 'Father of American Football'[67] Among these important changes were the introduction of the line of scrimmage, down-and-distance rules and of the legalisation of forward pass and blocking, a tactic that was highly illegal under the rugby style rules. Sport was fostered in young men as an essential tool for developing masculinity. Violence was not seen as an unfortunate side-effect – it was inherent and essential.

As one of the most prominent of the American Muscular Christians, Theodore Roosevelt believed that there were beneficial properties to American football's violence, as long as it could be reasonably managed. He was an avid sports fan and saw football as a way of revitalising a weakened and unmanly population who he deemed physically and mentally unprepared to defend themselves and take the world stage.

What is a pitch but a stage? When Benjamin Robinson was put in a different position to the one he usually played, in a team a man short, and asked to play on, would he not have felt the spectators watching him? Would he have understood his role, that of the boy learning the skills to become a man? Learning to 'take hard knocks without malice',[68] as said Bryan Mason – a desirable trait in possible future leaders. Rugby players deliberately and consistently put themselves in harm's way on behalf of others – on behalf of the team and in its common cause. This is what soldiers also do. A journalist, Mick Cleary, wrote in the British broadsheet the *Daily Telegraph* in 2013, after a young, unfancied England defeated Ireland in Dublin: 'These are no mere kids who need the roar of a Twickenham crowd to encourage them to puff out chests. These are guys for the trenches.'[69]

There are many comparisons to be drawn between soldiers and athletes, among the harsh and deadly demands of warfare and the thrill from a full-bodied contact sport like rugby. Both enable male camaraderie bonding and friendship, a heady mix of machismo and brotherhood. Both are aspirational, both follow a set of rules, both require an ability to keep going under severe stress, their successes dictated by a willingness to sacrifice personal glory for the good of the team. They even borrow language from each other – an abundance of military terms that have been adopted by sport – *blitz, bomb, formation, red zone, blow away.* Both also experience CTE and traumatic brain injury, the two most at-risk groups prone to neurodegenerative disease.

The Muscular Christians celebrated the body and the spirit in equal measure, which becomes problematic when considering the impact that violent pursuits can have. As David Titterington writes, 'The inevitable degeneration of the body implies a resulting degeneration of the spirit – a spirit which was supposed to be eternal, transcendent, and unchanging.'[70] In elevating the spirit through violent pursuits, you inevitably degenerate it. And what place does an incapacitated body have in a world of heroic men? Not a cherished one.

Men are gods, until they're not.

***

'My calendar tends to run immediately before the match, and then after, everything else tends to get lost,' Karen tells me, an explanation for the tangential way she has pieced back together Benjamin's story. She was slightly reluctant to speak to me in the beginning, wary of being misquoted or of her son's story somehow becoming skewed. It's happened before. The press are hungry for the story at first, hungrier still for photographs.

The image I had seen of Benjamin, the closely cropped photograph of him in his rugby kit, Karen calls his 'PR Photograph'. It would appear everywhere following his death. It's a good photo. He is smiling, looking straight into the camera, and he looks older than his 14 years.

'I would say, just thank God you're a handsome young boy because it would make for an ugly poster, son!' Karen says with a laugh. 'I just have to take it like that and go, yeah, OK, you're a good-looking kid. And it's just as well 'cause your face is everywhere!'

She pauses. 'I guess it's the dark side of the humour that maybe gets you through some things.'

The story of Benjamin's injuries and death amassed media coverage across the world – primarily in England, Ireland and the US. Karen and Peter's words, though, have been taken out of context, photographs of Benjamin snatched from Facebook accounts, not always maliciously but often without the prior knowledge of the family, meaning that every time a new photograph would emerge it knocked them back, more so when the dialogue around his death was solely focused on his athleticism and his love for the game.

'I think people get caught up in [the fact that] he's a fit, healthy, strong boy playing rugby. He's just passionate about it. And you know it's like a testament to his character and I'm going, "No. Can we just back up a bit because rugby does not define my son?"' Karen's tone is firm. Benjamin was not the poster-perfect rugby star. He was a 14-year-old boy, a loving son, a brother. He adored his family and the time he got to spend with them. He loved football, FIFA and Doritos.

★★★

Approximately thirteen months after Benjamin was initially laid to rest, a second burial was required. Benjamin's brain had been retained for pathological testing but with the tests complete and no formal date set for the inquest, the family had to apply in writing to the coroner's office for the return of the organ. She obliged, which is unusual.

Once again, Karen placed personal items and family photos with her son. This second service was conducted by the family's minister and was strictly private. The words 'Vibrant, Awesome, Loving' are inscribed on Benjamin's headstone.

It would be later that year, in September 2012 that the first inquest would take place. It lasted for five days with representatives from the Ulster branch of the IRFU (Irish Rugby Football Union) arriving on the fifth day, when it became apparent that the referee, who had been trained by the IRFU, was giving evidence without any legal representation. The Ulster branch had asked for a delay so it could prepare a report. The inquest was postponed.

'You expect people to give you answers,' Karen comments. 'And when you come out of an inquest with more questions than answers, it did seem as if we were up against not only the rugby authority, but the Education Board and the coroner's office, [too].'

Prior to the inquest taking place, they hadn't had legal representation, they were asking their own questions and lots of them. As former police officers, they knew how investigations worked and felt dissatisfied with the way things were going. So they hired a solicitor, which was fortunate because the school had hired a barrister. The inquest was to consider whether Benjamin had been concussed in an earlier tackle before he collapsed at the end of the match. The family had been told that Benjamin's injuries were the result of a one-off collision, and a 'freak accident' by doctors and representatives from the Ulster branch of the Irish Rugby Football Union. Peter recalls that a nurse had declared that Benjamin had more chance of being hit by lightning. But a pathologist found that Benjamin had three brain injuries, and it was probable that they had all been inflicted in that one match.

The consultant neurosurgeon at the Royal Victoria Hospital in Belfast told the family's solicitor, Mr Gabriel Ingram, that there were a number of witness statements left out from his report as he found the statements very challenging to piece together in a clear-cut way.

'It was a horrendous, emotional time for all involved – human nature, things get mixed up in terms of chronology and what was said,' he added.

What he did say, however, was that it would have been 'impossible' to know whether Benjamin had a concussion during the match and therefore should have been taken off before the fatal collapse.

The man in the sheepskin coat, who Karen recalled so vividly that day, was a senior doctor, unofficially in charge of first aid at the match. His own son was playing for the opposing team that day. Commenting later on whether he would have done anything differently following the first tackle Benjamin was involved in, he said:

> For this to have happened was a shock at the time and I am not sure what I would have done differently . . . if I had said he has to go off the pitch, they [the opposition] might have suspected I was doing it because he was a good player and wanted rid of him. I would not have been able to examine him with a degree of objectivity.

He also declared that Benjamin was back on his feet by the time he approached to examine him, and the doctor had no further concerns.

Peter and Karen strongly suspected that the school had been told not to admit anything by their lawyers, which meant that the version of events they were hearing at the inquest was very clinical and varied from Karen's recollection of that day.

It's not unusual for us to remember things differently – finding one single truth in any situation is virtually impossible – but neither parent had expected the school's version of events to be so different to their own or that of Benjamin's teammates, who, as Peter Robinson remembers, were given the toughest time by the school's barrister.

One witness from the match counted the seconds that Benjamin was lying on the ground before holding his head, just as Karen had recalled. He details that once back on his feet, Benjamin had asked him what the score was and if they were winning. The boy responded, 'Keep your head in the game.' In his statement he remembers Karen being on the pitch, the referee blowing the whistle and declaring that Carrickfergus had won. It was only later in the changing rooms that they were told that Benjamin had a concussion and had been taken to hospital.

The school's barrister challenges the witness that they couldn't remember events from so long ago.

'Do you agree that it can be difficult? Looking back?' they are asked.

The boy states that the memories are vivid in his head. For obvious reasons. And goes on to detail that he always checks to see who is lying on the ground to see who would be able to come on for them if they are out of play.

'I check for my teammates,' he said. 'I'm just making sure that my fellow players are OK.'

The boy is pressed further by the barrister about specifics, timecodes, whether or not he has taken notes on what previous witnesses have said.

It's an uncomfortable listen.

It is alluded to by the barrister that perhaps those memories aren't his and perhaps he colluded with other teammates before speaking to the police, since they didn't all make a statement straight away. He says that he did speak to teammates 'because we were all struggling to get through it', but not about speaking to the police.

The barrister continues by asking why an initial statement hadn't been made, to which the boy responds that the teammates were asked for statements very soon after the incident occurred, 'And none of us were really in the mood or in the right frame of mind for doing so.' He continues, 'And we were told that if you saw anything significant, that you should make a statement. We all talked about making a statement and we thought that there was no point in us making the statement at the time, because we thought it was clear what happened.'

The barrister says, 'So it was explained to you by, I presume, your principal at the school? How important it was – if you had seen anything important – to make a statement?'

The witness agrees, but states that at the time they didn't think that anything they had seen would be important because they knew that other people were making statements.

'And we thought that ours would just be the exact same as theirs.' He says, 'We didn't think that there would be any confusion in what had occurred.'

There is a childlike naivety to this statement and I remember that, at the time, these were 14- and 15-year-old boys who had just lost their friend and teammate.

The cross-examination is relentless. At the end of the questioning, Mr Ingram, Karen and Peter's solicitor, steps up to ask the witness if there was anything he saw that would suggest Benjamin wasn't OK. The witness details Benjamin's balance being off in the second half of the match, though he didn't put it in his statement as he didn't think it was relevant. There are no further questions.

The coroner, Suzanne Anderson, had said 'the frailty of the human memory when recalling traumatic events' meant that 'many of the witnesses were confused regarding timings'.

But then there was the video.

A police officer on the case had given Peter a video that was taken by the opposing team, the Dalriada School. They would often film their matches so that they could see where improvements needed to be made. Initially, in an act of kindness, the officer had handed it over so that Peter could see his son running about again. He tells me he made himself sick watching it. The police hadn't considered the video as evidence.

'I was watching it over and over again, sometimes until four in the morning, when everyone else had gone to bed ... every time there would be something new that I hadn't seen, something else I hadn't spotted.' He had the video slowed down and a screenshot with Benjamin circled clearly so there was no room for doubt.

The video was played in court on 3 September 2013. It's a particularly difficult listen given that it is Peter Robinson who steps up to narrate the final moments of his son's life. He begins by apologising for the late submission of the DVD.

'I couldn't go over the DVD. I just couldn't go through it again,' he tells the court. 'So, I put it off as much as I could.' But then he goes on to say that he had been frustrated by certain points of evidence throughout the inquest that had been contested. There is an objection from the courtroom that the coroner acquiesces.

'Just get on with the DVD for the moment if you don't mind,' she tells Peter.

Beyond Peter's voice, you can hear the film play out: the boisterous spectators in the background as well as the boys on the pitch; words of encouragement and instruction provide the backdrop for his testimony – 'bring it left, bring it left' and 'go on!' can be heard, encouragements of play, a reminder that, first and foremost, before the tragedy that unfolded, this was a game being played by children.

The first half of the match recorded on film went by without any major incidents involving Benjamin aside from the body tackle Karen had seen on her arrival. He already had a split lip and broken gumshield by this point, Karen remembers, but this collision was discounted because it wasn't shown in the video despite being in both her and the Coach's statements. The ferocity of play in the first half was enough for her to want her son taken off. I wonder if perhaps she knew; we've all had that foreboding feeling in the gut that tells you something bad is going to happen. Because after approximately one minute of play in the second half, Benjamin was involved in a heavy tackle, which led to the team coach coming onto the pitch to check his 'level of consciousness'.

Approximately four minutes later, he was involved in another heavy tackle, which resulted in him lying motionless on the ground for a short time, and which caused the Dalriada player to be taken off the pitch as he had sustained a knee injury. Benjamin's team coach came again onto the pitch. The coach had told the coroner that Benjamin had got up on his own, but the video clearly shows Benjamin being helped to his feet.

Benjamin had accelerated hard into the tackle. He appears to be out cold before he even hits the ground. Normally when you're falling towards the ground, you have your arms out to protect yourself, but his arms were by his side, his head taking the brunt of the fall.

'Benjamin was unconscious for a split second after that tackle, before he hit the ground,' Peter says. 'That's the only way I can explain how his body hits the ground like that. From then on, he keeps holding his right temple, with his right hand,' Peter says, 'throughout the remainder of the match, he's holding his right temple, with his right hand.'

Peter Robinson accepts that there is a grey area as to whether Benjamin was concussed from the tackle as he hit the ground, 'but lying motionless, grabbing, clutching [his] head, confused, not aware of the play of events . . .' He pauses, then continues, 'I, having played rugby myself, I definitely think this is the tackle . . . that does the damage.'

The video also showed the Dalriada player who Benjamin had tackled struggling, which is testament to the force of the impact. He can be seen bent over, looking towards Benjamin; the coach checks his neck and head.

'If you can imagine, this instance happened basically at the start of the second half. So, he's played, more or less, a full half, with the results of this tackle,' Peter says.

What was most telling was Benjamin's reaction as he was lying on the ground surrounded by rugby boots that are still in play.

'It's not a normal reaction for a rugby player,' Peter says. 'Everybody knows you protect your face. You lie in a ball. He's lying on his back with his hands on his head like that. That's no protection.'

Benjamin can be seen in the video hobbling around; seemingly disorientated, he repeatedly walks over to the sideline, continuing to hold onto the right side of his temple. He has a strange smile on his face. The coach approaches him often. Karen knew something wasn't right but she had witnessed her son being assessed and checked and allowed to play on. She had seen the coach moving his fingers from left to right in front of Benjamin's eyes at the match.

The video also shows Benjamin talking to one of his teammates, who, when questioned at the inquest, said that Benjamin had told him that he couldn't remember the score, and, at the sideline, his sister's friend told Karen that Benjamin couldn't remember anything. At one point Benjamin goes over to speak to his coach who insists he cannot remember what the conversation was about, but he knows that it wasn't about a head injury.

In the end, it transpired that Benjamin was checked for concussion three times during the match, and each time he was allowed to play on. There was a final stoppage close to the end of the match, the one Karen knew instinctively was for Benjamin. The video captures him knocked out on the ground for the final time. Witnesses at the match had said that Benjamin made a tackle, stood up, then collapsed backwards.

After the final hit, you can hear someone telling the person filming the video to turn the camera off when it's clear that he isn't getting back up. He never woke up.

Neither team were shown the video until the inquest. Something that Peter Robinson felt was detrimental to determining the events of the day,

'I know the numbers of the two players involved, for the Dalriada team, in both incidents, of the severe tackles,' Peter continues in the courtroom. 'I just don't understand why this footage couldn't have been shown to the kids to refresh their memory – Dalriada as well – and they could have come forward and said, "Yes, I was involved in that tackle, this is how I got injured. This is how … this is where Benjamin hit me. This is how the tackle panned out." Because this, this isn't a version, this is fact.'

The coroner agrees with Peter, telling him that the video is 'actually better than a witness statement in many ways, because this is … nobody can dispute this whereas statements can get confused'.

She asks the courtroom if there are any questions and a ten-minute break is agreed. 'All rise,' the usher says and there is incomprehensible chatter as the courtroom adjourns, but crying can be heard before the inquest recording cuts.

Peter calls it 'the perfect storm' – the series of events that meant his son, who would be in his twenties now, was left with multiple and ultimately fatal brain injuries from playing school rugby.

There were no questions when the court returned following the video.

The coroner speaks instead, stating that she has found the video evidence to have been extremely useful in ascertaining the chronology of events, 'Unfortunately, but understandably, given the frailty of the human memory when recalling traumatic events, many of the witnesses were confused regarding timings,' she says.

She continues. 'I'm satisfied from the evidence that he had sustained a concussion as a result of one of the heavy tackles in the first four minutes of the second half. During the rest of the match, he [Benjamin] continued to play enthusiastically and to display no immediately obvious physical signs that anything was amiss. Unfortunately, however, neither the team coach, nor the referee were made aware of Benjamin's neurological complaints, and he continued to play.'

As if it was somehow up to Benjamin, the victim and the one person who couldn't defend himself that day, to look after himself on the pitch. But Karen would still argue that the signs were there.

There is the Standardised Concussion Assessment Tool, or SCAT as it is commonly known, which is a card that lists the nine 'red flag' symptoms of a concussion. These symptoms are double vision, burning in the arms or legs, severe or increasing headache, seizure, loss of consciousness, deteriorating conscious state, vomiting, increasingly restless, agitated or combative and neck pain or tenderness.

The SCAT makes it clear that if any one of the symptoms has been detected then the player should be safely and immediately removed from the field. This is written in a bright red font to amplify its urgency.[71] It can very easily be found online and downloaded immediately.

The coach had testified that he had field tested Benjamin on three occasions during the match.

But the pocket SCAT or SCAT 2 were applied by neither the coach, Mr Kennedy, nor the referee, Mr Brown. During their evidence, both said that they were playing with what they refer to colloquially as 'rule-of-thumb tests' that they picked up over the years, essentially, using common sense. Mr Brown also confirmed that he had gone through the remainder of the 2011 season, and 2012, without any knowledge, again, of the pocket SCAT regulations.

The cards are not issued as standard, but they are available online to download and print for every rugby coach. It was put to the referee by Karen that he did not have knowledge of the guide that could be downloaded and read by anyone. He was asked if it was possible that Benjamin's concussion had been missed because of the 'antiquated methods applied'.

But he could not say for sure if the concussion had been missed.

When asked about the fact that the SCAT guidelines and regulations do not contain a warning about fatality – in fact, they do not contain the word 'death' at all – the medical director of the Ulster branch, Dr Michael Webb, said he thought that it was OK since if a non-medical person is doing the assessment and they suspect a concussion, it's clear that they should refer the patient for urgent medical attention. 'The onus would then be on the medical professional to know about those, and medical professionals will know about the risk,' he said.

He is challenged then by Mr Ingram, who reiterates that the absence of the word 'death' from the form could mean that parents, coaches or referees may not know that it could be a viable outcome. That without the reference, a layman would have no idea.

Dr Webb repeats that the risk is so very, very small.

He is then asked if he knows who Barry O'Driscoll is, a former international player who sat on the RFU medical committee for many years. He does. He is asked if Mr O'Driscoll is still in employment. He says he is not. When asked why, Dr Webb acknowledges that Mr O'Driscoll was uncomfortable when the 2011 guidelines came out around suspected concussion, which included the IRB sideline assessment bar.

The sideline assessment bar was designed to be a support for recognising sports-related concussions and to document clinical endpoints that may assist a qualified health professional in their return-to-play decision making. O'Driscoll had said in a *Daily Mail* interview that, 'In the five-minute test, the medic asks the player four or five questions when they are back in the dressing room.' He had said, 'They then have to stand for 20 seconds with one foot in front of the other without falling over. If they are able to do that, then they will ask them, "How do you feel?" That's ludicrous because at the top level these guys are real warriors – they are never going to say, "Can I stay off?"'[72]

The solicitor, Mr Ingram, told Dr Webb that O'Driscoll felt that rugby was trivialising concussion.

'He was uncomfortable with that,' Dr Webb agrees. 'And that's why he resigned from the post. He felt that if a player came off the pitch, they should stay off the pitch.'

Mr Ingram agrees. 'They are sending these guys back onto the field, and then to the most brutal arena. It's ferocious out there. The same player who 18 months ago was given a minimum of seven days recovery time has now been given five minutes.' Mr Ingram says, 'There is no test that you can do in five minutes that will show that a player is not concussed. It is accepted the world over. We've all seen players who've appeared fine five minutes after concussion or injury, then vomiting later in the night. To have this as acceptable in rugby, what kind of message are we sending out?"

'I think, when you're doing that assessment, it's difficult,' Dr Webb says. 'Sometimes when you're sitting, watch the pictures at home, for the doctor who's on the pitch, things happen so quickly and out of your line of sight, and it happens so quickly, so what you see is very different from what we see on a video. So, to defend some of those team doctors, the assessment is very, very difficult.' He affirms that there is no way that any player who has a concussion should stay on the pitch. 'That's a complete no brainer,' he says and repeats that the assessment is the most difficult one they do and that it's not getting any easier.

Mr Ingram goes on to say that 'the pocket SCAT 2 was recommended so that coaches, team managers, administrators, teachers, parents, players, match officials, and healthcare professionals associated with rugby teams, educate themselves using the IRB online training programme. So really, anybody connected whatsoever to rugby.'

Dr Webb adds parents and grandparents to the list, telling the court that parents can go on there and log on – considering it a good exercise for everyone to do.

'But it seems that the problem is that nobody, or very few, are logging on. And the message is not getting out there,' is fired back at him.

He acknowledges that that statement is probably right and gives an example from the perspective of a rugby coach: 'I got an email from the Ulster branch about the Pocket SCAT. So, I got that email as a coach, OK, and my fellow coaches at the team would have got that email. So, they've been given the information. But if I ask, you know, I know from talking to them, that they're not aware of it, because it's just such an information overload and it's how we get that message to people so that they take note of it, and they act upon it.' He says, 'How do we do that? That's the secret of all this. But it's not easy.'

There is a slight pause before the solicitor asks, 'Even with the death of a 14-year-old boy on a rugby pitch and months, years after that, would you agree that the message is still not getting out?'

'I don't think the message is where it needs to be, with as many people as it needs to be,' is the reply.

Mr Ingram states that the headmaster of Benjamin's school, along with the coach, Mr Kennedy, had later written to the chairman of the schools committee with serious concerns about the way concussion was being treated by the rugby profession and about the lack of advice given to coaches of school-aged players concerning the issue of concussion.

'I firmly believe that information of this importance needs to be disseminated to students in a more coherent manner. I also expressed the belief that a concussion clinic or seminar should be included in all underlying coaching courses run by the IRFU in future,' Kennedy had said.

It also details his concerns that in the months preceding the death of Benjamin Robinson the meetings were poorly attended, and not compulsory at this time.

'I wish it had been better attended is my answer to that,' Dr Webb says.

When questioned again about the danger of death not being included on the SCAT, he would later go on to list the benefits that sport brings in terms of recreational exercise and sociability, and the difficult task in balancing that against what he describes again as a very, very small risk.

'So, it's delivering the message that, you know, yes, it's potentially serious. But, actually, the risk is small. We don't want to alarm people so that they give up on sport because of something that is very, very rare,' he says.

But he also acknowledged that it was controversial as a subject because the numbers are so small.

It was put to him that perhaps it was fair to say that the literature on the subject also says that many of the cases were being misdiagnosed as something else, when in fact they were second impact syndrome.

Dr Webb agreed. 'I suppose that's right,' he said. 'And I suppose you're only going to diagnose it if you know about it, aren't you? So that would be a fair comment.'

The coroner ruled that Benjamin had died of 'second impact syndrome' (SIS), which occurs when the brain rapidly swells following a second concussion before symptoms from an earlier concussion have subsided. The second blow does not have to be concussive. A partial blow is enough to exacerbate the swelling, which is why it is essential to remove a player from a match as soon as the first signs of concussion are detected. If this is not done, the outcome is fatal.

The coroner's conclusion made Benjamin the first diagnosed case of second impact syndrome in Northern Ireland. The coroner found that Benjamin was concussed in the first four minutes of the second half, and that 'unfortunately neither the team coach [n]or the referee were made aware of his neurological complaints.'

Following the hearing, the IRFU issued a statement in which it expressed its 'deepest condolences' and stressed that 'injuries of this nature are highly unusual in rugby'.

The term 'highly unusual' does Benjamin Robinson a stark disservice. Concussion has been the most common injury in English professional men's rugby since 2011, with incidence rising an average of 1.2 times per thousand hours every season since 2002.

Second impact syndrome and ultimately death are the outcome of the injury, they are not the injury itself. But even the outcome is not rare, there are other young players who have died as a result of brain injuries from playing the sport. Rowan Stringer in 2013 and Lily Partridge and Sarah Chester in 2015. Those are the ones that made the news and yet the game continues to rage on every week in schools up and down the country.

'The only thing "highly unusual" was that it just wasn't managed,' Karen says, meaning the concussion protocol. 'It wasn't recognised for the killer that it can be. Concussion is a brain injury.'

The coroner, Suzanne Anderson, states that Benjamin had passed the tests that were carried out by the team coach to check his level of consciousness more than once. But there are no tests for children.

In 2017, A Child SCAT5 was introduced that detailed a symptom evaluation rather than the post-concussive symptom scale, and contained a health and behaviour inventory with a validated list for children and parents. It included red-flag signs and symptoms for early detection of mild traumatic brain injury (TBI). But this was much too late for Benjamin.

I think it's important to emphasise that until 2017, the rules for concussion protocol were built for professional players, men. It is also important to emphasise that SCAT is not a diagnostic tool, it is a recognition tool that determines what care – medical or otherwise – is required when an athlete is displaying verbal or physical signs of a concussion and the emphasis is to remove them immediately.

If in doubt, sit them out. And again, neither the coach nor the referee were aware of SCAT.

'Everyone in the inquest that day knew that there was no test for children,' Karen told me.

The coroner finished her closing statement by saying that there were indeed lessons to be learned in the case of Benjamin Robinson and stated for the court that she would be sending a copy of the findings to the head of Irish rugby and the Minister for Education Mr O'Dowd, directing Karen and Peter to work alongside the Minister for Education to raise issues regarding education for children, concluding that though boys who are playing rugby 'should be honest about having an injury, their teammates should be aware of looking for injury and parents also.'

Karen and Peter would go on to produce an information leaflet that would be distributed across all schools in the province that was publicly launched in 2014. It outlines what a concussion is in simple sentences so as not to be misunderstood, it also details the visible and audible signs of concussion to look out for, a return to school and play protocol, how teammates could look out for each other and the red flags to look out for. The word fatal is on the front of the leaflet. That was important. There is also a cut out concussion recognition tool with the words 'recognise and remove' in capital letters. Inside it also very clearly, and in capital letters, gives the direction that any athlete suspected of having a concussion should be removed from play immediately.[73]

A leaflet would be released in Scotland first, where Peter lives and where he would lead the campaign to improve education about concussion across Britain. Scotland's cabinet secretary for education, Michael Russell said at the time that Karen and Peter have been instrumental in ensuring there is 'a clear message to schools and sports clubs that concussion should be taken seriously and that anyone suspected of sustaining such an injury should be immediately removed from play.'[74] Peter directs me to a survey that was done in the lead up to the campaign with staff at 171 Scottish schools. It found that 30% of respondents would allow a player with suspected concussion to return to play.

On the back of the leaflet is the photograph of Benjamin, his PR photograph as Karen calls it and the sobering warning that 'his death could have been avoided had someone been able to recognise the signs of concussion and removed him from the game'.

'This child is our son Benjamin,' Karen tells me 'who was caught up in a chain of events which led to his untimely death. His death could and should have been avoided,' she reiterates.

Peter agrees. 'There should have been a chain of health and safety procedures in place, one that included players, coaches, referees and parents. If just one link in that chain had worked as it should have, Benjamin's concussion would have been spotted. He would have been removed from the pitch and he might have survived,' he tells me. 'It wasn't an accident – it was totally preventable.'

It went from Benjamin not wanting to let anybody down to Benjamin being let down catastrophically. The family are still left with questions.

To them, it feels like the inquest was a missed opportunity to reevaluate and reform the safety of the game from the very top down and to enforce crystal clear protocol to stop a similar chain of events from happening again. Instead, it felt like the waters had been muddied, that Benjamin had been blamed and it was left to them to make it right.

And yet sport remains a huge part of their lives. Their children still play football. They are the first to recognise the enormous benefits of sport too, but they also know the unimaginable consequences if correct protocol and safety procedures are not implemented, and information isn't distributed. They have taken it upon themselves to ensure that it is.

'We've had people saying, "Well, we can't stop the game every time somebody gets a blow to the head because it ruins the flow of the game." I would rather ruin the flow of the game than ruin a family's life,' Peter says. 'I don't ever want to hear about another Benjamin Robinson. Because then it really was for nothing.'

And I wonder who could argue with that? Who could honestly say that the sacrifice of a life is worth the flow of the game?

It's a word that comes up a lot, sacrifice, but who decides what that sacrifice is, and for what cause? Ultimately, it depends on whoever is making the rules.

'Jesus the teacher had become Christ the competitor . . . From the pulpit, preachers prayed for a winning season, striking their sermons with so much athletic symbolism that they sometimes sounded like commentators on TV sport broadcasts.'

— David Titterington[73]

Chapter Four

The Triumph of the Human Spirit

It wasn't until I had travelled hundreds of miles from home in London to Dhaka, Bangladesh, to make a documentary in 2016, that I had my own spiritual sports awakening.

Dhaka is the financial, commercial and entertainment capital of Bangladesh and yet despite this, over four million people experience poverty in some 5,000 slums across the city. We were focused on one in particular, Korail, a slum of approximately 200,000 people, and home to many of Dhaka's garment workers and their families. The workers were mainly young girls with dubious birth certificates that allowed them to legally (and I say that in its loosest term) work within the factories to support their babies.

We were shooting *The Forgotten Girls of Dhaka,* a television documentary and radio programme focusing on the girls living in Korail, who had been taken out of school and married off to much older men, only to be abused and later abandoned, either pregnant or with babies. They were effectively babies themselves, none of them older than 15. At the time I was torn between a subject matter that was difficult and devastating, and a setting that was alive and vibrant.

Upon arrival in Korail, we travelled down a rust-coloured road lined with vendors selling fruit and stirring steaming broths in large pots over open fires, their wares laid out on tables. Kids whizzed past on bikes, their limbs folded over handlebars, two or three riding together at a time. We were met by a kaleidoscope of colours at every turn, burnt-orange dirt tracks, washing lines strewn with bright cloth, the rainbow river of women and girls wandering to work wrapped in headscarves and long skirts.

We had already collected a trail of people behind us and as we pulled up to unpack the van, faces appeared in door frames and windows, around corners and on the top of the corrugated tin roofs. Smiles and eager eyes, full of intrigue and excitement. As we meandered through the myriad of houses, the Pied Piper allure of our cameras and pale skin would gather more smiles and more eyes.

By the time we had started rolling, there were hundreds of faces patiently waiting and watching. This would happen every day and though there was never really silence in Korail, there was a tremendous sense of peace. The call to prayer from the local mosques would glide across the surface of the water that separated the slum from the city, emerging from the banks like a gentle breeze wrapping itself around the stir of crickets, the swooping of birds and the hustle and bustle of life, filling the sky with an unfamiliar song that would start to feel comforting as the days wore on.

Most of our trip was spent shooting early in the morning so as to avoid the stifling heat. Until, later in the week, as is the nature of the filming beast, we had overrun late into the afternoon. Dusk was settling in, the call to prayer had long rippled out across the water. The heat had slightly subsided and the sun had painted the sky in a violent red. Soon it would darken, making way for the moon, barely visible as it was above the city's smog.

We wrapped up and, as night fell, the power suddenly cut out across the entire slum, plunging us into darkness.

'It happens,' our driver offered casually, as if to reassure us. 'Sometimes it just goes out. There's only one generator.'

With phone lights we began to make our way back through the maze of bamboo and corrugated-iron-sheet homes towards the van. It felt different that night – the place we had got to know during daylight, now an unsettling stranger. We struggled to get our footing, taking numerous wrong turns and, for the first time all week, I realised it was completely silent, save for a distant rumbling none of us could quite put our finger on.

Perhaps most unnerving of all was that while we had spent the week surrounded by people, tonight there wasn't a single person to be seen – all the houses were empty. As we moved closer towards the main road, we caught flickers of light above us, sets of eyes watching us from the roofs; the faces of young men suddenly became illuminated by one bright light we could make out towards the end of the track. They were smiling, the ominous rumble revealing itself as the cheers from a crowd.

The light was from a projector that was playing out an Asia Cup cricket match between Pakistan and Bangladesh onto a bed sheet that had been stretched across the dusty road and tied to phone masts and wires overhead. The projector was being powered by that one generator, usually reserved to provide for the entire slum. The projector itself was a generous donation from an affluent businessman in the city, our translator told us.

Our driver nodded his approval. 'Everyone deserves sport,' he said.

Every single inhabitant was here, gathered in the street, sat on top of the houses, on the roofs of cars, hanging out of window frames to watch the match. The air was electric. Kids were allowed to stay up late, eyelids propped up by excitement. We stood, taking it all in, shaking our heads with laughter at the absurdity of being the only people in the entire country, let alone Korail, that didn't know that this match was happening.

Bangladesh won that night: how could it not? Divine intervention, perhaps.

The following morning, we arrived at a scene of a young boy midway through a match with his dad, having fashioned a bat out of a chunk of wood, whooping with delight, drunk on hope and possibility as the ball collided with the bat, sending his dad skidding up the track with no chance of a catch.

'He's gonna win the cup one day! Why not? He's seen it!' our driver laughed. A father, son and the triumph of the human spirit. The true power that sport holds over people.

★★★

Dr Bennet Omalu is late for our first conversation. I'd tried contacting him through various media, including DMing through Twitter, to no avail. His secretary cut me off at the pass.

When we do finally manage to speak, in 2018, Dr Omalu said it was 'serendipity'. In reality it was more likely to do with the company I was working for and the founder who'd been seated, at his own request, next to the doctor at a charity function, who then contacted me afterwards to say he was very keen to work with him in some capacity. I explained I'd been trying and sent over a very tight, one-paragraph pitch and we were immediately introduced.

Dr Omalu is credited as a seminal figure in the discovery discourse around CTE in the NFL. His life was immortalised in the movie *Concussion*, with Will Smith in the starring role.

For most people, the port of entry to the subject, even to this day, is via *Concussion*, which spiked a search for 'CTE' on Google around the film's release.

It told Dr Omalu's story - how he tried to convince the authorities to act and create awareness among the public about the presence of CTE in American football players.

'I was so naive!' Dr Omalu exclaims. 'Will Smith teased me [about it]. He said, "Bennet, you're one of the naivest people I have ever met."' He is laughing now 'But . . . actually it was my naivety that propelled me to do what I did.'

Dr Bennet Omalu has many titles. He is a forensic pathologist, a neuropathologist, an anatomical pathologist, a clinical pathologist and an epidemiologist. He examines both living and dead people who've suffered all types of trauma and studies the patterns and distribution of disease in populations, and CTE has been ingrained in his life and work for decades.

He is a conflicting character, subject to constant scrutiny by both the sport and scientific communities. By his own admission, he credits struggling with depression as one of the reasons he discovered CTE in the Pittsburgh Steelers' player Mike Webster. A discovery that catapulted the disease into the spotlight.

He recalls, 'I was very socially bashful, and I had no social life. And I had such low self-esteem, so I spent so much time alone and that made me engage with relentless creative thinking. So, in that process I encountered football and began to wonder, since football was such a violent sport, why wouldn't the players suffer some type of brain damage? So when I met Mike Webster, I had that on my mind.'

The meeting Omalu is referring to took place in 2002, on his autopsy table, after Webster died suddenly, aged 50. Although it initially appeared normal, the doctor subjected Webster's brain to very extensive analysis, which confirmed that there was damage to the former NFL legend's brain, consistent with CTE. In bringing this to public attention, and while 'this historical evidence demonstrates that the long-term consequences of repeated head trauma in football players were recognised long before the explosion in media interest',[74] Dr Omalu helped to set in motion a chain of events that would cost the NFL millions of dollars, leading to questions about the rules of the game and also to the elevation of his own story to Hollywood property.

There is a dominant narrative in the US that describes overcoming a great challenge and becoming better and stronger because of it. Perhaps you know it. This is Horatio Alger Jr's 'rags-to-riches' story, prevalent in American culture. A Harvard-educated novelist and former minister, Alger wrote hundreds of short stories in the late nineteenth century that propagated the myth that anyone could work hard and become rich, a self-made man. Which ties into the idea of the American Dream.

That anyone can become something from nothing.

The stories that Alger wrote followed a few basic themes. The main character was either an orphan or runaway from a poor background, who had to support himself or his family. He would end up in some kind of situation where he would help someone and, in return, received money or a better job. The story – and message – were invariably the same: through work, perseverance and luck, you can get rich.

If there were two men who embodied this more than most, it would be Nigerian-born Dr Bennet Omalu, who came to the States and excelled through sheer hard work and determination, and the man who would open further doors for him, Pittsburgh Steelers' player Mike 'Iron Mike' Webster. Like many young athletes, Webster saw sport as his way out of a small town and an unhappy, violent and poor home. One of Webster's high-school teammates commented: 'Football was Webster's refuge from his gothic childhood, almost a matter of survival.'

So, Webster, like many of his peers, would do whatever it took to succeed. He played in the NFL for 17 years, and his success and tenacity were hard to match. His story isn't unique to sport. There is a fire that comes from having nothing and needing to escape. It propels you forward and is consistent with the rags-to-riches narrative present within the stories of a lot of heralded sporting heroes, Aaron Hernandez among them. Hernandez, whom Dr Ann McKee examined post-mortem, grew up in Bristol, Connecticut and is often framed as the embodiment of perilous masculinity.[75] Shawn Courchesne notes that Hernandez's family 'didn't live in the best area of Bristol and they weren't wealthy', and asserts that '*obviously* if you live in an area like that there are going be [negative] influences'.[76]

Hernandez's story is often trivialised in keeping with the Great American Success Story narrative – overcoming a traumatic childhood, and rising to sign a multi-million-dollar contract extension with the New England Patriots two years into playing for the team. Like Webster, he was presented as the phoenix rising above the ashes of his circumstances. It fitted with the idea of the American Dream, that sport was an escape, a way out. And once you've had a taste of that, you'll do anything to keep it. I'll come back to Hernandez shortly.

***

One of American football's notorious drills is called the Oklahoma drill, named after Oklahoma's coach Bud Wilkinson, who popularised it in the 1940s. It involves head-to-head contact, putting players across from each other in an enclosed space as they ram into each other like bulls until someone is thrown to the ground or put out of play. You can see it for yourself on YouTube in countless videos. It's fast and the ferocity is shocking, but it's the sound of the helmets colliding that stays with you. Like the crack of bones.

Sometimes, the drill would become a public spectacle, with the same players repeatedly pitted against each other as fans and fellow players watching the practice would gather, cheering them on. It was likened to a modern-day gladiator fight.

In an interview with *Frontline*'s Jim Gilmore on 29 March 2013, former NFL agent Leigh Steinberg, who once represented NFL stars such as Troy Aikman and Steve Young and organised conferences to educate his clients about the risks of concussions in the 1990s, was asked about the use of violence and the effect of its glorification. He said,

What's a more powerful image in football than a violent hit? And it began to be a subject that was glorified. There were actual shows showing the hardest hits. NFL Films marketed different DVDs which were *The Hardest Hits*. The actual logo of *Monday Night Football* is two helmets hitting together. And it became part of the popular jargon. You know, 'He knocked him silly'; 'He knocked him to the moon'; 'He rung his bell.'[77]

Webster was tenacious during the Oklahoma drills, using the same strength that earned him the nickname 'Iron Mike'. He had a reputation for durability that led him to play through injuries in an era when head injuries were considered just part of the game. Webster's centre position is one of the most exposed and unprotected positions on the football field. One that is particularly exposed to blows from offensive linemen. In the 1970s defensive linemen used a technique called the 'head slap', in which they would begin their rush by slapping the centre and other offensive linemen on the sides of their helmets to disorient them,[78] though this was banned in 1977. That said, there are still instances of players taking slaps to their helmets; sometimes this isn't a violent strategy to assist play, but rather to congratulate a player for their game.[79]

The range of symptoms Webster suffered from was vast – he had dementia, depression and acute bone and muscular pain; he was on a cocktail of drugs most of the time including Prozac, Ritalin to help him focus and ease his depression, and Elderpryl, which is primarily prescribed for those suffering with Parkinson's symptoms. He had become homeless, struggled with money, and was living out of his pick-up truck or in bus stations, refusing to accept 'charity' from friends or family. His memory was impaired, and he suffered daily headaches that, as he once told his doctor, felt like 'the top of his head would blow off'.[80] He would use a taser to ease his back pain and he had superglued his teeth in. In 2002, aged just 50, Iron Mike died of a heart attack. It was a tragic ending to what had become a tragic life.

And although his brain injury had been acknowledged in the 1990s, it was only when Dr Bennet Omalu came along that 'Iron Mike' Webster's brain injury would stand for something, causing debate in the NFL and further afield into player safety. There are few conversations around CTE that don't involve Webster or Omalu, both as historical and cultural touch points, seminal moments in this ongoing debate. To say it's a messy story would be an understatement. There was the threat of potentially being kicked out of the United States. He had become something of a celebrity himself, a role model, which despite his natural bash-fulness, he seems to have stepped into with ease.

Dr Omalu is 20 minutes late to our first meeting. My phone finally buzzes and I can hear that he is driving as he apologises profusely for getting 'caught up' – and by 'caught up' he means that he was stuck doing a post-mortem on a young Black man who had been shot.

Outside of his work on CTE, Dr Omalu has, as I've said, many roles. It was he who conducted the independent autopsy of Stephon Clark in March 2018. A young Black man, Clark had been shot by two Sacramento police officers who claimed they believed Clark was pointing a gun at them despite the fact he only had a mobile phone on his body. On 30 March, Dr Omalu released his findings, stating, 'You could reasonably con-clude that he received seven gunshot wounds from his back.'[81]

His report, which also found that one of the bullets was likely to have been fired while he was already on the ground, was controversial, not least because there were discrepancies between Dr Omalu's report and the one produced by the county forensic pathologist, Dr Keng-Chih Su. The latter indicated that Clark had been shot once in the front of the left thigh, three times directly to the side and three times in the right side of the back.[82] On 2

March 2019, Sacramento County District Attorney Anne Marie Schubert announced that her office would not be filing criminal charges against the police officers involved in Clark's death.[83]

'I'm sorry, I'll be 15 minutes! Long day!' Dr Omalu shouts cheerily before hanging up.

There's no denying that Dr Omalu is captivating. When he does speak, his voice booms as if he is delivering a sermon, then swiftly drops to a whisper. He speaks as though he is address-ing the masses at a rally, not just me, on the end of a phone 5,000 miles away in London. He gives you his all, one minute his voice soft so that you have to lean forward to concentrate, the next booming. It's an impressive technique, one I've often seen adopted by politicians or actors on stage, lowering their pitch so you have to give them your undivided focus. And there are parts of our discussion that feel rehearsed, performative even, and that thought doesn't sit well with me, but then again Dr Omalu has had to answer the same questions over the past 15 years.

Following his discovery of CTE in Mike Webster's brain, Dr Omalu published a paper in the esteemed medical journal *Neurosurgery*.[84] It was the first case of CTE ever to be found in a former NFL player and, as a result, sent shockwaves across the football community.

Dr Omalu had been certain that he would be providing an invaluable service not just to medicine but to the NFL, that they would welcome his discovery with open arms.

'I thought they were gonna come and embrace me and say, "Motherfucker, you're such a hero,"' he had said in an inter-view with journalists Mark Fainaru-Wada and Steve Fainaru for *League of Denial: The NFL, concussions, and the battle for the truth*.[85]

This would be the making of him, and something that would improve and save the lives of many. He felt it was his duty, not just as a scientist and physician, but also as a Christian, to announce his findings and to formulate a hypothesis. After all, this wasn't a brand-new discovery. There existed anecdotal evidence and hundreds of papers pointing to the relationship between head trauma and neurodegeneration in athletes, as far back as Martland and the boxers in the 1920s. It was, however, the first time a finger had been publicly pointed at the NFL where CTE was concerned.

'I was naive,' he repeats flatly to me.

Dr Omalu grew up in Nigeria; he didn't understand what the NFL stood for or that American football was a major component of American life. In other words, he didn't quite realise the immensity of what he was getting involved with.

'I was a total ignoramus! A total buffoon of football. I did not know anything about football!' he bellows, adopting the tones and exaggerated temperament of the preacher mid-sermon once more. 'I didn't know what a quarterback was. I didn't know what a touchdown was. All I knew was that this was a game and people wore helmets to intentionally slam their heads into one another!'

Before Dr Omalu's discovery, in 1994 the NFL commissioner, Paul Tagliabue, created an NFL-run Mild Traumatic Brain Injury (MTBI) Committee as a result of a number of high-profile concussion-related retirements and injuries within the sport. Tagliabue described concussions as a 'pack journalism issue' during a panel on the future of sports. 'On concussions, I think [this is] one of these pack journalism issues, frankly ... There is no increase in concussions, the number is relatively small ... The problem is a journalist issue.'

In order to shape the NFL's concussion research[86] around the committee, he would hire Elliot Pellman, a rheumatologist and the New York Jets' team doctor, who had described players as 'like steelworker(s) or soldier(s)' and concussions as 'an occupational risk'.[87]

Following a spate of high-profile injuries, in 1997, the American Academy of Neurology established guidelines for athletes returning to play following a concussion. They recommended that where loss of consciousness had occurred, players be 'withheld from play until asymptomatic for one week at rest and with exertion'.

Despite the increased prevalence of concussions and players including Steve Young, Chris Miller and Troy Aikman being sidelined (or leaving the game altogether), in an interview with the *Chicago Tribune*, Pellman would state that the MTBI Committee's studies have found that brain injuries in football are relatively minor.[88]

After four years of keeping close track of head injuries, Pellman claims the numbers have remained 'remarkably the same' throughout the league. He said there are about 180 'incidents' per year of mild traumatic brain injury. 'We're talking the majority are minor injuries,' Pellman said.[89]

In an interview with the *New York Times* in 2000, NFL doctors and members of the MTBI Committee criticised the 1997 guidelines, stating they were not supported by enough research. 'We don't know whether being knocked out briefly is any more dangerous than having amnesia and not being knocked out,' said neurologist Mark R. Lovell. 'We see people all the time that get knocked out briefly and have no symptoms,' he added.[90]

However, in 2004, MTBI Committee member Lovell, along with Karen M. Johnston and James P. Bradley, authored a paper after the concussion management guidelines suggested that athletes with mild (grade 1) concussions may be returned to play if asymptomatic for 15 minutes. The purpose of the study was to assess the utility of a current concussion management guideline in classifying and managing mild concussion.

They concluded that:

> Athletes with grade 1 concussion demonstrated memory deficits and symptoms that persisted beyond the context in which they were injured. These data suggest that current grade 1 return-to-play recommendations that allow for immediate return to play may be too liberal.[91]

The MTBI Committee would regularly publish research that appeared to be on the fence regarding the breadth and severity of concussions and how they were attained.

In publishing his report on Webster and CTE, Omalu inadvertently became a whistle-blower. Members of the NFL's MTBI Committee swiftly called for his research to be retracted, damning Dr Omalu's claims. They cited the description of CTE as 'completely wrong' and 'a complete misunderstanding of the relevant medical literature' in an open letter written to the editor of *Neurosurgery*.[92]

None of the authors of the letter were neuropathologists with the exception of one neurologist, Dr Ira Casson.

Their argument is summarised in *League of Denial*.

> They made two primary arguments: that Omalu et al. had a case that didn't meet the criteria for CTE and that there wasn't enough clinical evidence showing Webster was mentally impaired. They insisted Omalu's findings met only one of the four standards necessary to call this CTE, even though Omalu and his colleagues had never claimed this was identical to what was found in boxers. The NFL doctors suggested that the clinical history on Webster was essentially useless because it had been limited to a few phone

calls with family members. They pointed out that Webster had no history of concussions or any indications that he had ever left a game because of a blow to the head.[93]

And yet Webster had been diagnosed with brain damage resulting from multiple head injuries he sustained during his football career much earlier than Dr Omalu's findings – in fact, while Webster was still alive and had submitted a report for disability benefit. The details of which are laid out in a court report released from the United States District Court, D. Maryland, Northern Division when Sunny Jani, the administrator of the estate of Webster, sued the Bert Bell/Pete Rozelle NFL Player Retirement Plan and the NFL Player Supplemental Disability Plan (collectively, 'the Plan') for wrongful denial of benefits under the Employee Retirement Income Security Act of 1974 ('ERISA').[94]

The initial report included an examination from Dr Fred Krieg, a clinical psychologist, who found after examining Webster that he was 'totally and permanently disabled as a result of brain damage received during his career as a professional football player'. Krieg observed that 'although it is [to] Mr Webster's advantage to have "done poorly" on this evaluation, he really tried throughout the interview to make himself look as good as possible, covering up certain information'. Although Webster told Dr Krieg that he was self-employed after his retirement from football, Dr Krieg reported that 'he really can't substantiate any kind of gainful employment'.[95]

There was also a report from Dr Jonathan M. Himmelhoch, a board-certified professor of psychiatry at the University of Pittsburgh who serves as the Director of the Research Affective Disorders Clinic at the Western Psychiatric Institute. He was also of the opinion that Webster was totally and permanently disabled, with a 'traumatic or punch drunk encephalopathy, caused by multiple head blows received while playing center in the NFL'. [96]

'The Plan' also required Webster to undergo a medical examination by a neurologist of its choosing, Dr Edward Westbrook, who also found Webster to be totally and permanently disabled as a result of multiple head injuries, and that his disability began in March 1991.

The case text details that on 5 November 1999, the Plan informed Webster that he had been approved for total and permanent *degenerative* disability benefits. [97] Which means that it was acknowledged, though the benefits were limited. Contrary to the collective conclusion of the experts, including one selected by the NFL, the NFL found that Webster's disability did not exist when he retired from the sport.

NFL spokesman Greg Aiello later emphasised to the press that the retirement board is independent, and that its decisions 'are not made by the NFL or by the NFL Players Association'. [98]

It feels strange to me, then, that there was pushback from the NFL in regards to Dr Omalu's paper when Webster's brain damage was widely acknowledged. Though this didn't deter Dr Omalu and his co-authors, who countered the attempt at retraction with a second paper. [99] This time they studied the brain of another deceased NFL player: Terry Long, an American college and professional football player who was an offensive lineman in the NFL for eight seasons during the 1980s and early 1990s, playing for the Pittsburgh Steelers.

Long had been found unconscious in his home aged 45 and later died: his cause of death was determined as suicide by drinking antifreeze. As with Mike Webster, Dr Omalu found that Terry Long had also suffered from CTE. [100]

Dr Joseph Maroon, the Steelers' team neurosurgeon who joined the MTBI Committee in 2006, told the *Pittsburgh Post-Gazette* that Dr Omalu's conclusion about Long's suicide possibly having been the result of depression caused by head injuries during his career in football was 'fallacious reasoning'. He added: 'He could have had a head injury that wasn't reported before football. He could have had a fight. He could have had a head injury . . . And that's why I'm saying it's so speculative.'[101]

Omalu also examined the brain of Andre Waters, who had shot himself in the head in 2006.[102] Waters, who'd played for the Philadelphia Eagles and Arizona Cardinals, was considered one of the hardest hitters of the NFL. Omalu determined that Waters' brain tissue had developed chronic traumatic encephalopathy (CTE) and degenerated into that of an 85 year-old man with Alzheimer's disease, caused or hastened by the numerous concussions Waters sustained playing football.[103]

It was Chris Nowinski, a former Harvard football player and professional wrestler, who'd been fearless in his participation of sports, who initially approached Omalu. He loved American football: he loved the game, he loved the physicality. By his own admission, he loved the physical challenge of it. He played with ferocity: he wanted to impress, wanted to be tough, which meant he never admitted to having a concussion in his entire football career.

He justified that by saying that in football everything always hurt, that pain was just weakness leaving the body. In his 2006 book *Head Games,* which examines the concussion crisis in American football, Chris writes: 'I was told: if it ain't bleedin', it ain't hurt. Suck it up. Take off your skirt, Sally. That was the culture I loved.'[104] This attitude is something he carried on into his professional wrestling career with the WWE, years later.

'The willingness to play hard is an interesting construct,' Chris tells me, 'because in a sport like American football, you need to have a willingness to play hard to succeed. Like, it's an incredibly painful game.'[105]

On the one hand, he thinks it actually made him better and tougher, more prepared for what he does now and the life he has had. But that work and life has also been very painful. 'And you just learn to accept it and keep pushing, and the problem that exists with the culture of playing through pain is that we never talked about the brain.'[106]

Chris's career was over as result of the injuries he sustained, but also as a direct result of his 'play-on' attitude. He spent his mid-twenties struggling with severe post-concussion syndrome. He details a five-year headache and three and a half years of sleep walking that would involve breaking windows or smashing his nightstand if he wasn't heavily sedated.

Nowinski was worried for his future and sought treatment with Dr Robert Cantu where he finally realised the long-term impact of his injuries and the real dangers of concussion. His concussion education prior to meeting Dr Cantu was next to nothing – afterwards, it was a very different story.[107]

Now he's not only concerned for his future, one that he's almost certain could involve CTE, but also, his subsequent work on concussions and their effects caused him to have grave concerns for other players, particularly young people, and about how the NFL handled the subject and injuries.

It was Nowinski who called Andre Waters' family to get the former player's brain. At the time it was unprecedented for a researcher to do this, but the Waters' family wanted to know what happened to Andre and why he had changed so much in the last five years of his life.[108]

'When you have the responsibility of actually possessing somebody's brain,' he said in an interview with *Frontline*'s Michael Kirk, 'you really treat it with the utmost respect, because you have a piece of them. And you have probably the most important remaining representation of who they were.'[109]

Dr Omalu called Nowinski to confirm that Waters had suffered from CTE.

Dr Omalu later examined former Steelers' offensive lineman Justin Strzelczyk, who, after leading the police on a high-speed chase through central New York in 2004, collided at 40 miles per hour with a tractor trailer. It exploded on impact, killing Strzelczyk instantly. Again, Dr Omalu found CTE in Strzelczyk's brain.[110] Dr Ronald Hamilton of the University of Pittsburgh confirmed Dr Omalu's announcement: 'If I didn't know anything about this case and I looked at the slides, I would have asked, "Was this patient a boxer?"'[111] According to the *New York Times*, Dr Kenneth Fallon of West Virginia University also confirmed his assessment.[112]

The NFL didn't back down though. Two years after Omalu's first publication on CTE, the NFL were producing safety pamphlets for players stating: 'Current research with professional athletes has not shown that having more than one or two concussions leads to permanent problems if each injury is managed properly.'[113]

Prior to this, the MBTI released research that stated that:

current attempts to link prospective grading of concussion symptoms to arbitrary, rigid management decisions are not consistent with scientific data. We believe that if one insists on grading concussion severity, the best way is retrospectively, on the basis of how long it actually takes the player to become asymptomatic, with normal results on neurological examination. It is the recommendation of the NFL's Committee on Mild Traumatic Brain Injury that team physicians treat their players on a case-by-case basis, using their best clinical judgment and basing their decisions on the most relevant, objective medical data obtained.[114]

The CTE findings were intended to improve standards, not just in American football, but in every other contact sport. Rugby, ice hockey, boxing, wrestling, mixed martial arts, lacrosse, football – every sport where players could suffer repeated blows to their heads. That was the objective, that the NFL could lead by example.

'We are constantly looking to improve ourselves, aren't we?' Omalu's voice is low and I catch myself leaning in once more. I know where he's going with this. If we did something a certain way in 1950, and then in 2005, for whatever reason, we discovered that it might not be good for us, common sense dictates that we would change how we do it, surely?

'Exactly,' he responds, when I tell him this. 'Like smoking.'

It's a sad comparison, but an absolutely valid one to make between the way that the tobacco industry treated the causal link with cancer and how repetitive head injuries and neuro-degenerative diseases are viewed. In court, you cannot prove a causal link, but what you can prove is a strong association between smoking and lung cancer, just as you can prove a strong association between repetitive head injuries and early-onset dementia and other neurodegenerative illnesses.

***

The brains arrive fresh in cardboard boxes. They are wrapped in a series of plastic bags and packed in a Styrofoam cooler. When they are taken out of the box they are weighed; all the external surfaces are photographed and then a series of dissections are made. The brain will be cut into sections.

'We'll freeze half of the brain, snap-freeze it at minus 80, and we'll store that in freezers for scientists that want to look at molecular or biochemical studies. Genetic studies will require frozen tissue,' McKee said. The other half of the brain is preserved before being dissected and photographed for a whole series of microscopic slides, so that analysis and diagnosis can be made.[115]

'It's sort of a Sherlock Holmes type of mystery,' Dr Ann McKee tells me. 'You have a patient who comes in with peculiar symptoms and then you want to know the reason why there's a lot we don't know about the brain.'[116]

As a clinical doctor, she became interested in the brain. She went from internal medicine to neurology and, during her training, had a lot of exposure to neuropathology. 'I realised that's what really fascinated me – I wanted to pursue neuropathology so that I could understand the biological basis for people's symptoms.'

Before CTE, McKee was very involved in Alzheimer's disease and neurodegeneration with a focus on tau protein for '20 odd years'. One of the cases that came to her was that of a world champion boxer, Paul Pender, who had been part of McKee's Alzheimer's study in 2003.

She found his brain fascinating, with an unusual pattern of the tau pathology.

McKee had to find out if something like this had been described before. 'We needed more of these examples to really make something of it. You can report a single case, but it won't be a very important study. But if you can find a series of them, and really understand what this disease is, you can make an important contribution,' she told *Frontline*'s Michael Kirk.[117] She was looking for another boxer when she came across the report by Bennet Omalu on Mike Webster. 'I remember seeing it and thinking, *That's exactly what I saw in this boxer.*'

Ann Mckee's formal introduction to CTE would come through Chris Nowinski.

Since the diagnosis of Andre Waters, Chris Nowinski and his team had begun to acquire the brains of more deceased athletes for study. They came into the possession of the brain tissue of NFL player Tom McHale, who died aged 45 of a drug overdose, as well as that of an 18-year-old high-school student who'd died ten days after suffering his fourth concussion. Both were diagnosed with CTE.[118]

McKee analysed Tom McHale's brain. He had previously been a lineman. Nowinski later said in an interview that 'we didn't assume everybody who had a bad outcome had CTE. But we figured there was a chance, because he was a lineman for so many years, and because he did change, because usually successful Ivy League family men don't become drug addicts overnight. So, there was a question worth looking into.'

McHale's family received an initial call from Bennet Omalu about doing a study, but after speaking to Nowinski, they thought it would be worth having two study groups and agreed to give Tom's brain tissue to both parties.

There was extensive damage to McHale's brain and the pathology was just like Paul Pender's.[119] But the boxer was almost 30 years older than McHale, who was in his mid-forties.

From that point on, there was no going back. They had a duty of care to players, former and current, to share their findings. The NFL at this point were still downplaying CTE, saying it wasn't a big problem, attributing the damage to other factors including steroid, alcohol and other substance abuse, and citing that there may be other confounding factors in terms of the genetics that they simply didn't understand.[120]

In May 2009, McKee was invited to present her findings to Dr Ira Casson, co-chairman of the MTBI Committee at the time, and members of the committee at the NFL headquarters in New York. Dr McKee later claimed to *Frontline*: 'It was like, "Oh, the girl talked. Now we can get back to some serious business."'[121] Dr Henry Feuer, then a committee member, responded, telling *Frontline* that Dr McKee's research did not indicate a specific cause for CTE and could not show the prevalence of the disease, given that her findings were based solely on case studies.[122]

'I just have a problem,' he said. 'Ann McKee, she cannot tell me where it's starting. We don't know the cause and effect. We don't know that right now. We don't know the incidence. [...] She was seeing only those that were in trouble, and we know that there are thousands roaming around that are not having problems.'[123]

'Of course,' McKee tells me. 'Sport is [worth] billions of dollars, billions and billions of dollars, and a real identity and cultural feature of many of our countries, so [CTE is] not going to be something that's an easy sell.'[124]

McKee's attitude towards the game has changed. 'I can't say that I'm a big fan of the game anymore. It's changed. It's hard for me to watch, but I really want to keep the players safe. I want kids to be able to play sports, soccer and, you know, participate. I think it's very important to physical and social wellbeing to be able to play sport. And I just want to make sure that we are doing things when we're playing sports that are keeping individuals healthy for the rest of their lives. Not subjecting them to something that will reduce their ability to think before they're even out of their adolescence intentionally.'[125]

Or worse, I think.

'I'm determined,' she says, 'determined, to do what I can to eradicate [CTE].' She sighs. 'And it's hard, I'm tired. Because we've been trying to push a rock up a hill for decades now and we've made progress, but it seems slow in coming and meanwhile, you know, getting brain after brain in ... it's going to require a lot of intellect from very many corners of the earth to really eradicate this disease.'

In a 2017 study published in *The Journal of the American Medical Association*,[126] McKee and her fellow researchers examined the brains of 202 former American football players from all levels of the game. They found that 110 out of 111 of those who played in the NFL had CTE. In 2018, McKee made *TIME*'s 100 Most Influential People list because of her research.

One of the brains examined in 2017 by McKee and her colleagues was that of Aaron Hernandez, the former New England Patriots' player, and a convicted murderer. McKee said that at the time Hernandez's brain showed one of the worst cases of CTE she had ever seen in such a young person: he was in his late twenties at the time of his death. His brain was riddled with Stage III CTE. McKee told a news conference that 'individuals with similar gross findings ... were at least 46 years old at the time of death'.[127]

Hernandez had been serving a life sentence without parole for the 2013 killing of semi-professional football player Odin Lloyd when he died by suicide. Hernandez, who had always protested his innocence, did not raise CTE in his defence at trial.

McKee had stated: 'While I'm not going to connect the dots with his behaviour or difficulties during life . . . the frontal lobes – and his were very severely affected – are involved in problem-solving, judgment, impulse control, and social behaviour. The amygdala, which was affected in Aaron Hernandez as well, is involved in emotional regulation, emotional behaviour, fear, and anxiety.'[128]

The NFL responded to the research report, acknowledging McKee for her work, stating:

> We appreciate the work done by Dr McKee and her colleagues for the value it adds in the ongoing quest for a better understanding of CTE. Case studies such as those compiled in this updated paper are important to further advancing the science and progress related to head trauma. The medical and scientific communities will benefit from this publication and the NFL will continue to work with a wide range of experts to improve the health of current and former NFL athletes.[129]

As noted by the authors, there are still many unanswered questions relating to the cause, incidence and prevalence of the long-term effects of head trauma such as CTE, and the NFL stated their commitment to supporting scientific research into CTE and advancing progress in the prevention and treatment of head injuries. This included a pledge of '$100 million in support for independent medical research and engineering advancements in neuroscience related topics. This is in addition to the $100 million that the NFL and its partners are already spending on medical and neuroscience research.'[130]

They conclude with: 'The NFL deploys 29 medical professionals on the sidelines for each game. Working with the NFL Players Association, the league enforces a concussion protocol for players that has been instrumental in immediately identifying and diagnosing concussions and other head-related injuries.'

Today, the VA-BU-CLF Brain Bank, where McKee is director, houses 70 per cent of the world's CTE cases. Out of more than 1,000 brain donations, about two-thirds have tested positive for the disease, some in people as young as 17.

'I never forget that the brain is a human being. And the brain, to me, is a life,' McKee tells me.[131] She is an enormous advocate for sport and believes it's essential to a productive and healthy life, but is adamant that it has to be safe.

'CTE is a fact,' she says firmly. 'If you had the experience that I've had of young individuals in the prime of their life coming in with this devastating disease that has ruined them and led to their death in one way or another . . . ' Words escape her momentarily. 'I mean, I see this every day, and I listen to it every day.'

McKee feels she has a responsibility to speak for the players, players that went in for a dream and ended up broken. The psychological impact of CTE, not just on them, but their families, too, is immense.

The Concussion Legacy Foundation's story is widely reported, as are those of Bennet Omalu, Ann McKee and Chris Nowinski, but their interactions with the NFL are a microcosm of the much greater problem of sporting bodies' handling of CTE.

The NFL is the obvious starting point, one that at the time of beginning this investigation was the most documented and discussed – or, at least, most openly. But it could be argued that their position in the spotlight shielded other sports from accountability or awareness surrounding the issue – that is, unless you were willing to pull at the thread that, once unravelled, would extend the narrative from the American NFL pitches to Australian laboratories and on to the UK homes of Dawn and Laraine Astle, and beyond.

'How do you know who to trust?' I asked Chris Nowinski during our conversations.

'Oh, man, you don't!' he roared, his laughter drawn deep from the belly.[132]

'Beware of powerful sports associations. They will try to stop you.'
— Erik Matser, neuropsychologist[133]

Chapter Five

Media, Myth and Medicine

When I was younger we spent one Christmas along with a group of friends, renting a youth hostel in the Peak District. The teenage boys of the group had commandeered the only room with a small television and DVD player and would spend their evenings with the lights off, door firmly shut, making their way through the selection of action movies the house had to offer.

My stepsister and I would occasionally crack open the door to spy on them, the unmistakable heady mix of Lynx Africa and the sort of sweat that only five teen boys in a darkened, windowless room could conjure stinging our nostrils. We would stand very still, swallowing back our laughter so as not to be caught until betrayed by our own giggles.

'GET OUT! BOYS ONLY!' they would bellow from the shadows and we would scram, slamming the door behind us.

When I say I first saw *Gladiator* at 14, I don't mean the entire film. I saw *Gladiator*, or *the* Gladiator for a few minutes. We had heard a ruckus one evening, the clang of swords against a chorus of 'NO WAY's and 'AHHH's and 'OOOH's that intrigued us. When we entered, Maximus Decimus Meridius was sitting at the back of a cage surrounded by men about to enter the auditorium. He looked handsome enough to curb a giggle and keep two teenage girls from risking being sent away.

In one scene, Maximus is with his Master, Antonius Proximo, who is berating him for the seeming lack of flare to his killings, declaring that it's not a butcher the crowd want, but a hero. He reminds his gladiator that he is an *entertainer*.[134]

Maximus doesn't flinch, his eyes are fixed ahead and unfazed; armour is thrown to him and he's ready to fight.

We were gripped; so were the boys, who remained focused on the screen without so much as a heckle back at us.

Maximus, played by Russell Crowe, was the ultimate pin-up hero: he was strong, silent, gorgeous. You know how it goes: resigned as general, father to a murdered son, husband to a murdered wife and bought as a slave by Proximo in a North African market – which meant that ultimately, besides his looks and fighting ability, he had absolutely nothing left to lose.

He was Proximo's prized asset and would fight to the death. It was quite the performance, even watched through the gaps in my fingers. The squelch of sword slicing through flesh, the crunch of bones and the roars of masculinity were visceral and violent even without the visual. Soon it was over.

'Are you not entertained?' Maximus roars, flinging his sword skywards and sending it crashing into the Emperor's box. His eyes are wild, intoxicated on fear and victory.

'Are you not entertained?' he repeats, more loudly, arms outstretched, chest broad, circling his audience, taking in each and every face, a real showman. 'Is that not why you are here?'

He releases a second sword, sending it clattering to the ground and spits where it lands. In the room, the boys grunt in approval as the crowd on the screen goes wild, chanting, fists pumping, cheers rippling like a Mexican wave from the rows and rows of hungry fans nestled within the colosseum. He is little more than a performing animal to the crowd. Here is their champion. Here is their show.

***

You can always tell the people that have been fucked over. They're the ones that agree to talk straight away, that don't edit their words; it's not that they're reckless, but they're not cautious either. They're not hiding. At least, not anymore. Australian neurophysiologist and adjunct professor Alan Pearce is happy to talk on the record. I was sent to Pearce via researchers who had been working with him. Another link in the chain.

Pearce's primary research focus is on sports-related concussion. He co-wrote a paper about Graham 'Polly' Farmer – the first Australian-rules footballer to be diagnosed with CTE.[135] Farmer died in 2019 at the age of 84, after a long battle with Alzheimer's, but was posthumously diagnosed with Stage III CTE following tests on tissue from his brain at Sydney's Royal Prince Alfred Hospital by pathologist Michael Buckland and his team. Pearce first had the idea to 'try the case', drafting the initial findings alongside Buckland and his team.

Alan Pearce was born in Perth, Western Australia and Polly Farmer had been a name he had heard a lot about as a kid, although Farmer had retired from Australian football by then.

'He had that legend-type status, like Jeff Astle, in that sort of league,' Alan tells me, 'and, you know, there's a freeway named after him!'[136]

I laugh. Jeff Astle had a bridge named after him. Primrose Bridge, in the heart of the Black Country, in England, has been known locally as Astle Bridge after the words 'Astle is King' were daubed on it to mark the striker's winning goal against Everton in the 1968 FA Cup final.

After the media reported that Polly Farmer had passed away after suffering from Alzheimer's, Pearce had said to Buckland that they had to get hold of his brain, and made moves to contact the family. Farmer's daughter and son hadn't actually ever thought it was Alzheimer's and were happy to donate his brain to science. Farmer had dementia for over 20 years: most people with Alzheimer's do not live for 20 years. The average person lives four to eight years after receiving the diagnosis.[137] The patterning of how his behaviour changed also wasn't necessarily in line with the symptoms of Alzheimer's.

The examination of Farmer's brain meant Pearce and Buckland's team were able to diagnose CTE.[138] They released a paper on their findings that also posed the question, why hadn't CTE come into the equation before?

'When someone presents with a number of symptoms, a lot of neurologists will quite happily say, "I just know it's Alzheimer's." So that's why we're trying to call for more post-mortems,' Pearce says, 'because in Australia, anyway, post-mortems of the brain are not done on a regular basis.'[139]

The news travelled fast and the story made frontpage headlines around the world. Pearce and Buckland held a press conference with 20 different media outlets.

There were those that challenged the diagnosis: Sam New-man, who had played with Farmer for four seasons on the same team appeared on Triple M's *The Hot Breakfast* with Eddie Maguire, and Luke Darcy, telling the radio hosts of how people tend 'grab a narrative and run with it'.

'I'm a little sceptical of where this is all headed,' he said. 'I wonder if the people who took brain samples from Graham Farmer took them from Muhammad Ali or Joe Frazier or any-one else who's been belted. I know it's a problem, but we get a modicum of truth in all these things and people exploit it. I have no idea if Farmer suffered from concussion but in the very long period of time, I knew him both on and off the field and, socially, I never noticed any ill effects from him playing our game. We all got knocked around a bit and I treat it with scepticism.'

I ask Alan how the Australian Football League (AFL) responded to his paper and it doesn't surprise me when he says there was initially 'complete silence'.

When I reached out to the AFL CEO Gillon McLachlan for comment I was quickly passed on to a spokesperson whose initial response was promising. They stated their confusion around Alan Pearce's claims of 'complete silence' surrounding Polly Farmer and said that the 'AFL certainly acknowledged the diagnosis of Farmer and have since encouraged former players to donate their brains to learn more about CTE, etc.', along with a promise of providing further information regard-ing the above, which never came.

There was a statement from the AFL in regard to Farmer, which came a day after the announcement. Pearce rattles through it in a monotone way about the concussion manage-ment policy having improved over the years and the players' health being paramount. 'The stock phrases,' he calls them. I can see why it felt like 'complete silence'.

Gillon McLachlan thanked Farmer and his family for donating his brain and for the learnings and medical fraternity they would get from it. 'Clearly, it's about prevention, diagnosis, and about research, and we'll continue to learn. The health and safety of our players is paramount and we'll continue to work with the medical fraternity and the experts in all those three areas to make sure our game is safe at all times.'[140]

As the public conversation increased, and it was clear that this story wasn't going away, there were more responses. More key figures in the AFL entered the discussion. AFL Players Association board member Scott Pendlebury publicly stated that the game has changed over the years when it comes to concussions and head injuries.

'One thing I can say in my time is that it's improved immensely. It used to be the whole thing about how hard you are and how tough you can be, after a big hit you get back out there and it was almost lauded, whereas now, if there's a big hit, guys are off, they're done for the game and most likely they won't be back the next week. I think the AFL and AFL Players Association, we're doing all we can, we're learning as much as we can to look after guys and in the past ten to fifteen years, that stigma's changed around the hard guy getting back out there to protecting the head and looking after guys as much as we can.'[141]

There were other statements from the AFL then and over the years. Reading them feels like a strange version of *Groundhog Day*, those stock phrases again that aren't unique to the sport either, far from it in fact, they can be found across the globe in different countries and from the mouths of different organisations.

The league later went on to say in a statement:

> As knowledge and understanding of concussion has increased, the AFL has strengthened match day protocols, changed the Laws of the Game to further discourage high contact, and has improved the identification of potential concussive incidents through the use of video. The AFL further strengthened the Concussion Management Guidelines for the 2020 AFL and AFLW seasons which reflects our ongoing conservative approach in managing concussions at the elite level. The AFL will continue to invest in research to better identify and manage concussion and other brain-related trauma at all levels of the game.

In 2019, there would be Danny 'Spud' Frawley, another former player and coach, who died aged 56 by suicide, by driving his car into a tree.

Nicknamed 'Spud' because he grew up on a potato farm, Danny Frawley played 240 games for St Kilda before he turned to coaching. He initially played as a forward but soon became a renowned full back. According to the AFL community club site, some of the key characteristics for being a good full back include having great body strength for one-on-one contest, an aggressive mindset in contested situations and a willingness to take the game on.

Australian football is often confused with rugby but the game is more fluid: players have much more freedom of movement, on a much bigger oval-shaped pitch. The balls are different too, though the ferocity with which the game is played is similar. There are collisions, impacts. It is as beloved in Australia as the NFL; it's the country's most popular sport: players like Polly Farmer and Danny Frawley are incredibly admired.

Frawley was well respected in Australia. He was the longest serving captain at St Kilda until 2014 when he was overtaken by Nick Riewoldt. He went on to commentate the AFL for Triple M, Fox Sports, SEN and the Nine Network, as well as work part-time as a defensive coach, and became an advocate for men's mental health, openly discussing his own struggles with depression that culminated in a nervous breakdown. The news of his death rocked the sport; people were beside themselves. If you look at any video clip of Frawley on YouTube, he's happy; he likes to have a laugh. He was a real campaigner for mental health – men's mental health in particular. And then, suddenly, he was gone. Frawley's diagnosis, at least, wasn't critiqued like Farmer's had been.

I wonder if the violence of his suicide somehow clouds the diagnosis, diverting public attention away from the root cause of what occurred. It reminds me of Aaron Hernandez, who Dr Ann McKee stated had one of the worst cases of CTE ever seen. Hernandez was convicted of violent crimes though, which were the driving narrative in his case, as we've discussed already. Media analysis has found that while CTE did not seem to play a factor in media depictions of the case prior to diagnosis, the diagnosis did impact how the case was reflected following diagnosis. He was a murderer – that's the label that prevails.[142]

And unlike Aaron Hernandez, who had a difficult childhood and supposedly struggled with drug abuse and a confused sexuality (though these claims are not grounded in anything concrete in Danny Frawley),[143] it is CTE that is listed as 'a potential contributor to the depression that Mr Frawley suffered for some years preceding his death'.[144]

The response to Frawley's death was one of great mourning – headlines reported the 'sad' and 'tragic' news.[145] There was an 'outpouring of emotion'.

In March 2021, St Kilda and Melbourne put on *Spud's Game: Time 2 Talk* – a celebration of the life and memory of the late Danny Frawley, which was also an opportunity to promote a national conversation around the prevalence of mental ill-health in the community.

They held a pre-game tribute to Frawley, including delaying the game by two minutes, to allow those watching to check up on their mates. Melbourne champion Garry Lyon addressed the audience, 'Whether you're sitting here in the stands or at home watching on the television, it's a time to talk,' he said. 'If you've got an issue at home, if you've got a problem, if you think there's something that needs to be said, we are encouraging tonight to talk – and that's what Spud would've wanted you to do.'

He noted that Frawley had three great loves – his family, his mates and to compete.

'And this time, right here, just before the game was starting, was when he was at his best, because he was standing alongside his mates and he was eye-balling the bloke across the line – and that was what he was all about,' Lyon continued.

Hernandez's death in contrast garnered 'mixed emotions' due, in part, to him being incarcerated at the time. It was reported that he died as he had lived – a mystery to everyone. But the descent and death of both men share a commonality, that we could never truly know what was going on beneath the surface. And, in both cases, no one appears to have seen it coming.

'And once we had Danny Frawley it was the same response. You know, the health of the players is paramount and we can't change what happened in the past, and all this other stuff,' Alan Pearce says.

Once again, the AFL were called upon to respond to the escalating situation. The official statement from Gillon McLachlan felt familiar. One catastrophic death from Farmer, and from a previous AFL statement.

> We have strengthened match-day protocols for the identification and management of concussion, we continue to change the Laws of the Game to discourage high contact and also moved earlier this season to change the Tribunal rules to more strictly sanction tackles that endanger the head. The ARC, which we introduced in the last year, has also provided another opportunity to identify potential concussive incidents through the use of world-leading video technology.
>
> The AFL further strengthened the return-to-play aspects of the Concussion Management Guidelines for the 2020 AFL & AFLW seasons which reflects the ongoing conservative approach in managing concussions at the elite level which then feed into community football.
>
> We continue to support further research being undertaken to assist us taking action, including by further rule changes, to protect the head and the overall health and safety of Australian footballers at all levels.

Unlike Farmer whose cause of death had initially been attributed to Alzheimer's, the post-mortem examination by Victorian coroner Paresa Spanos found that Frawley's pathology was low-stage CTE. There was nothing else. There was no Alzheimer's. Nothing at all that could confuse the picture.[146]

I find a series of black-and-white photographs of Frawley printed in the *Herald Sun*.[147] In one he is lying on the floor, one hand holding his head; the caption reads: 'Frawley lies stunned after being hit behind the play.' In another he is lying 'unconscious on the ground after a clash with Dermott Brereton in 1988'. In another he is being helped off the ground by trainers, much smaller than he is, his face distorted, eyes screwed tightly, mouth open as if he is letting out a cry. He looks in pain. A final image shows Frawley's side profile, having sustained a cut above his ear in 1989, his hairline matted with blood that has stained his cheek.

Frawley's death and subsequent diagnosis coincided with the clinicians and researchers from the Royal Prince Alfred Hospital NSW Health Pathology and the University of Sydney's Brain and Mind Centre, including Dr Michael Buckland, uncovering the first evidence of CTE in Australian rugby players.[148] The research was conducted on the brains of two middle-aged professionals who played more than 150 top-grade rugby league games each throughout their careers. At the time, Michael Buckland told the *Sydney Morning Herald* that it was the wake-up call they needed that Australian sports were not immune to the disease.

'I've been in this job for ten years and I would personally report 100 brains a year from a variety of sources,' he told the *Sydney Morning Herald*. 'We see all sorts of stainings when we assess anyone with any cognitive impairment and these changes I have not seen before. They're distinctive.'[149]

At the time the National Rugby League said that it would review the study's findings before making any detailed comment but said its approach to management of head injuries is based on global best practice.[150]

'The NRL has significantly increased its focus and investment in this area of player safety and will continue as an active participant in the work of the global sport community to advance the understanding and management of head injuries in contact sport,' it said.[151]

I have found that a lot of the official responses from the leagues tend to say very little in terms of action. There are promises made, reviews mentioned; they feel like holding pages to me. 'The more they can do that, the more they can continue without concern of litigation or people not wanting to play the sports,'[152] Pearce says. The last line he rolls out in a tone I have often come to hear throughout this investigation, one that lies somewhere between fatigue and exasperation as if to say, 'How are we still playing *this* game?'

★★★

Recent changes to the AFL saw a 12-day stand-down protocol introduced, which meant men and women would be required to sit out a minimum of one game in the event of a concussion, assuming regular fixturing, and potentially more depending on clinical symptoms.[153] Previous rules allowed players to return after six days (and therefore potentially play the week after a concussion). But Alan thinks players suffering heavy concussions should be sidelined for a minimum of 30 days.

He calls the protocol 'a PR campaign' and has publicly stated that 'these decisions are about being seen to do something rather than actually making sound decisions based on research or what is best for the athletes' health and welfare and in the long-term, in the game more generally'.[154]

Within the recent response I received from the AFL, they had offered to provide further information of their actions taken over the last ten years, particularly in recent years in the concussion space, noting that it would be a good starting spot as it would 'challenge some of the claims about what they have and haven't done' that I had put forward.

There was an offer of a Zoom call for clarity as well as official statements in regards to the series of claims that I put forward. But neither have surfaced.

Despite chasing, at the time of this book going to print, I had heard nothing more from the AFL representative.

***

Alan Pearce isn't afraid to speak up. I'm surprised there haven't been more repercussions for him; 'I mean, I've had my own personal problems . . .' he tells me. 'And that's why I do independent research now. So, it makes it a little bit easier that we're just running this without being under any auspices of any sport as such.'

He wasn't always independent. The 'problems' he encountered began when he was approached by the AFL who were offering to fund his research, if he would be happy to work with them. He wasn't surprised when they came calling in 2015: he had published a study on retired football players and concussion along with studies on amateur/non-retired players. The funding they were proposing would allow Pearce to replicate tests he had used successfully in a previous study of retired amateur and elite Australian-rules footballers in their fifties, using a technique known as transcranial magnetic stimulation (TMS), to measure brain activity and motor control.

He would be recruiting retired players with a history of concussion, from among 600 who had responded to an online AFLPA survey in 2014, which revealed that one-third had high levels of anxiety and depression. The terms were agreed.

It wasn't great funding, he admits, but it was one or two days a week, so enough to keep him going. He accepted it.

'Did you sign a non-disclosure agreement?' I ask him.

Alan's response is quick and unguarded. 'I had to. It was written into my contract and I needed the money.'[155]

Things became complicated quite quickly when the AFL advised Pearce that they would, in fact, be selecting the people he would test, which felt suspicious as it relinquished Pearce of control, despite the fact he had already developed protocols for his own testing.

The setbacks for him were only just beginning. It would be five months until the AFL would send across the first former player for the study. Pearce had expected to look at 200 players, knowing that a third of the 600 former players who had responded to his initial survey had complained about the ongoing problems of concussion. He alleges that he would have meetings with the AFL where parts of his study would be swapped in and out. 'It felt like they wanted parts of the research project, but not all of it,' he tells me. They had also decided that the neuropsychological and ophthalmologist testing would be done by other people and the results wouldn't be shared with Pearce, who argued that he needed all the variables to put it all together, because otherwise the key part of the research, the waveform activity that he was measuring using his technique, would have no context, essentially deeming it worthless. They concluded that that was OK.

Pearce says participants would come in and say they hadn't had previous testing, despite his insistence that testing was essential for this kind of research. It didn't make sense.

'And I'm like, you're kidding, right?' Alan says. 'So, I'm just trying to scratch my head, going, what? What's going on here?

And in essence I think they were just trying to completely undermine the research.'[156]

There would be more trouble for Pearce when a story about his 'ground-breaking' research was aired on ABC's *7.30*, which was described as the first time the AFL had ever studied the long-term effects of concussion. The reporter, Louise Milligan, stated that the research represented a 'significant shift in its attitude towards the long-term effects of concussion', since the AFL had previously been 'sceptical' about CTE.[157]

Shortly after the broadcast, on 12 October 2015, Pearce received an email from Associate Professor Paul McCrory, one of the leading members of the AFL's expert concussion group, asking if he had been granted permission by the University of Melbourne to both do the story and film in the lab. It was his understanding that this was non-negotiable if he were to undertake the work. The sign-off is short, instructing Alan to sort it out.

Alan was confused. He was adamant that permission had been granted, that he wouldn't have gone ahead if it hadn't been. He reiterated the steps that were taken to gain that permission. Two days later, Pearce received an email from Linda Denehy, the head of the university's department, requesting a meeting with him. He enquired what it would be about and her response was 'bad news'. That they did not have support for his contract after the conditions they had discussed were not met. She felt it was best he knew now.

The discussions that had not been met, Alan tells me, were 'doing no media'. Despite his insistence that Denehy had verbally agreed in a meeting with him later that morning that he had asked for her approval. Though this couldn't be confirmed. I put this to Linda Denehy but had no response.

A few months later, the AFL formed the view that Pearce's research 'was not delivering productive outcomes' and, therefore, the research wasn't continued. Pearce states again that due to the restraints that were put on him and the fact that essential elements were taken out of his control, the research he had done was worthless.

It is his opinion that Denehy was railroaded into letting him go, describing Paul McCrory as having an 'eminence that influences people'. In two days, the physiotherapy department had stopped the research, the lab was shut down completely and Pearce had to find somewhere else to go. The university later said that approval had not been provided for ABC to do the story, with Linda Denehy telling a reporter at the *Monthly* herself that she had decided that her department was unable to supervise his concussion research. Alan tells me that he was told while he had said nothing wrong or 'anti-AFL' in the story, it was 'factually incorrect' because the report did not say that the Florey were 'the world leaders in concussion research'. He says, 'I also know that they were in fact asked and turned an interview down.'

Alan later told journalist Andy Burns what had happened.

'I was very surprised when Alan emailed me and said that he was in trouble for having the crew come and film at the lab,' she said. 'He did not seem to me like the sort of person who would be a media cowboy or go off without permission and book a film crew to come to the lab.'

It is her belief that Alan thought he had firm permission from the 'higher-ups' and was 'blindsided when they came down hard on him for it'.

She tells me she found it even stranger given the context of the report, which was simply there to inform the viewer that this research was being done for the first time by the AFL and in her opinion, there was no cause of contention or secret information being leaked.

'Perhaps his only mistake was a bit of naivety about the sensitivity around the issue, a naivety that I probably shared at the time,' she says over email.

Andy Burns said that she had also emailed McCrory prior to the television report to ask for his expertise on CTE. 'And I recall getting a one-line response along the lines of "I am not going to talk about that".'

The abruptness took her by surprise, especially since this was his area of expertise.

'And you know, then I had to wonder what sort of hornets' nest I had walked into.'

I also reached out to McCrory in regards to the television interview and Alan Pearce's claims, but heard nothing.

McCrory is a expert in the concussion field, carrying heavyweight titles including Associate Professor of the prestigious Florey Institute of Neuroscience and Mental health, as well as being a consultant neurologist, general physician and sports physician with particular expertise in the area of traumatic brain injuries. He is considered a global leader in the field of sports concussion and CTE. In 2021 he was listed in the 250 top researchers in Physical Education and Sports in *The Australian*'s *Research* magazine.[158]

My initial introduction to Paul McCrory was a video on YouTube of a lecture he had given at the Florey Institute in 2016 entitled 'The Concussion Crisis: Media, Myths and Medicine',[159] during which he states that the problem in the NFL has been grossly overblown and argues that the dangers of concussion in the NFL are not nearly as serious as some reports have led the public to believe. He accuses the media of presenting 'oversimplified views' and remarks that not all hits cause brain damage but 'certainly shakes things up'. He has questioned the significance of NFL-related findings from Ann McKee and Boston University and claims that those complaining of ongoing problems as a result of concussion were '50- and 60-year-old people who have got worries for all sorts of reasons'.[160]

It has been widely reported for years that he has a reputation for challenging research that establishes a link between repeated blows to the head and neurodegenerative disease, claiming that 'this CTE thing is not what it's cracked up to be'.[161] Ninety per cent of people, he says, got better in a couple of weeks. In essence, the entire lecture casts doubt on whether the CTE 'story' is true.

The Florey Annual Report for 2015–16 backed this up by stating, 'Paul remains sceptical of the simplistic view that the number of concussions suffered in a sporting career results in long-term brain damage.' He is quoted as saying: 'It's really not a scientific statement. It's more of a belief system.'[162]

It's not the first time he's suggested the science around CTE is the stuff of make-believe. In 1999 his paper 'The eighth wonder of the world: the mythology of concussion management' was published. For clarity, the Merriam-Webster Dictionary defines 'a myth' as an unfounded or false notion, or a person or thing having only an imaginary or unverifiable existence.[163]

The conclusion of the paper is as follows:

In this era of evidence-based medicine the challenge for sports medicine is to develop a scientific approach to this common clinical problem. It has been 1,000 years since the first clinical description of concussion by the Arabic physicians and the time has come to replace management myths and clinical anecdotes with medical science.[164]

A paper from 1999 may feel a long time ago, before the substantial evidence of CTE had mounted. But all evidence suggests this was a view that stuck. In June 2015, a paper titled 'Neurodegeneration and Sport' was published listing Paul McCrory as an author.[165] In the abstract it states:

The recent interest in concussion in sport has resulted in significant media focus about chronic traumatic encephalopathy (CTE), although a direct causative link between concussion and CTE is not established. Typically, sport-related CTE occurs in a retired athlete with or without a history of concussion(s).

While many of these athletes have a history of exposure to head impacts as a part of contact sport, there is insufficient evidence to establish causation between sports concussion and CTE. It is likely that many of the cases with neuropathological findings represent the normal ageing process, the effects of opiate abuse, or a variant of frontotemporal lobar degeneration.

In February 2015, just months before his June paper, McCrory released an article on second impact syndrome (SIS) titled 'Does "Second Impact Syndrome" Exist?',[166] as part of *The Oxford Handbook of Sports-related Concussion*, which was being developed in 2014.

Second impact syndrome is a condition that is believed by some people to be a consequence of recurrent sports concussion. The only evidence to support its existence is anecdotal and, if it does exist, it is rare. The fear of this condition has driven the promulgation of concussion management guidelines and, more worryingly, the recent trend towards government regulation of the clinical management of concussion in the United States. Diffuse brain swelling following a single head injury, a well-recognised condition, is more common in children than in adults and usually has a poor outcome. It is posited that the so-called second impact syndrome simply represents diffuse brain swelling mistakenly attributed to repeated concussion.[167]

Three months after Benjamin Robinson, the 14-year-old boy who died in 2011 of what the coroner ruled was 'second impact syndrome', a 17-year-old female Canadian rugby player called Rowan Stringer sustained a fatal brain injury despite prompt medical therapy. According to a study published in the *Canadian Journal of Neurological Sciences*, 'The cause of the massive brain swelling was initially unknown. An inquest revealed Rowan's text messages to friends describing symptoms from two prior, recent rugby brain injuries, likely concussions, within five days of the fatal blow.' It also confirmed the diagnosis of 'second impact syndrome'.[168]

Debating the existence of SIS is dangerous and I would argue reckless, especially if you are at the helm of an international concussion in sport group like Paul McCrory is.

But I didn't get a chance to argue; McCrory did not respond to my request for an interview about his work or the group.

The group has organised the major consensus meetings in the field and was originally brought together in 2001 by the International Ice Hockey Federation, FIFA, the FIFA Medical Assessment and Research Centre and the International

Olympic Committee Medical Commission. Read those names again – they are all sports associations with millions to billions in turnover. The main objective of the group was to 'understand, as completely as possible, what actually takes place when severe blows to the head occur'. It was their hope that 'with the information learned, we can begin educating our athletes with the goal of eliminating concussions in all sports'.[169] A large part of the group's job was to advise on how to manage the issue of safe return to play of concussed athletes, and they would hold conferences 'to provide recommendations for the improvement of the safety and health of athletes who suffer concussive injuries in ice hockey, rugby, and football (soccer) as well as other sports',[170] and to establish 'a single "concussion in sport" definition, at a time when many disparate definitions existed'.[171]

Their Berlin conference of 2016 produced a highly influential statement.[172] The outcome statements for each conference are important, often cited by coaches, athletes and trainers at the very highest level when making key decisions, so much so that they have been dubbed the 'Bible' of sports concussion and medicine and are adopted and referenced by sporting bodies worldwide.[173] Outside of sport, if you have ever suffered a concussion, it's likely that the treatment you've received was influenced by their statements.

According to the latest study published in 2016, 'a cause-and-effect relationship has not yet been demonstrated between chronic traumatic encephalopathy and sport-related concussion or exposure to contact sports'.

Critics from across the global news media are raising concerns about the panel's affiliation to sports federations and the strong influence they may have on any scientific research.

This can be seen in articles published by the Dutch newspaper *NRC*, the *Guardian* and the Canadian Broadcasting Corporation.[174]

In 2020, CBC news in Canada analysed the résumés of the 36 expert panellists from the 2016 statement and found that 32 have, or have had, 'connections to organisations in sports where concussions are a major issue'. These are readily available, either on public websites or in the conflict-of-interest statement that is published at the bottom of research papers where you would be hard-pressed to find one that doesn't indicate an author's affiliation to a sporting body, whichever side of the fence you sit.

'[T]hose relationships include employment, consultancy work, research grants and expert witness testimony. Many of the links existed at the time the statement was written,' journalist Jeremy Allingham reported.[175]

In his article, he quotes Chris Nowinski, who said that the consensus included 'some of the greatest [CTE] sceptics that are out there'. Nowinski said, 'There are certainly a great number of concussion experts who I respect on that paper,' but he emphasised that 'concussion experts are not CTE experts'.[176]

On the first day of that 2016 conference, those in attendance were discouraged from communicating to the outside world via social media. There are some tweets that include screenshots of attendees startled by the dramatic move for a medical conference that was hardly MI5. I put this to Paul McCrory as well, but again, heard nothing back.

It begs the question, in the realm of concussion, what exactly is there to hide?

'I mean, put it this way,' Alan Pearce says. 'I think the AFL's last television deal was probably nearly three billion dollars. So, you can see what sort of money has been thrown around here. So, something like concussion comes in and shows that the players are being brain damaged; they're at risk of dementia or even dying on the field. You know, that could be bad for business,' he claims. These claims were put to the AFL, and they did not respond further.

It's not the first time I've heard this, I tell him. He assures me it wouldn't be the last. 'It's just a whole rabbit warren you end up falling down,' he offers with a shrug.

Meanwhile the players played on, and the conversation in the media ground to a perceptible halt.

'I think it also comes down to the branding of those sports,' Pearce says.[177] 'So, again, it's very similar around the world. It's the same with commentary. "Oh look, he's coming off the field. He's going to be looked at. He's got the best doctors in the world looking after him. He will be fine!" So, the average person in the public listens to that and goes, "Ah, you know what? He's going to be fine."'

Commentators are often well-known ex-premiership players who the spectators know and trust, so when someone trusted says that the AFL have got the best doctors in the world – we've got nothing to worry about, have we?

I'm reminded of this watching a 2020 Euros match – England vs Poland when captain Harry Kane had taken a mighty hit to the head from a player's elbow and is on the floor for close to ten seconds. The collision isn't acknowledged by the commentator but Kane's 'lockdown hairstyle' is.

'And what we get is constant rhetoric that comes throughout, just their own advertising and branding and communication, but also through television and radio. It means that the conversation is almost one-sided because very rarely is the average person sitting there reading scientific papers, so they don't have the capacity necessarily to question it,' says Pearce.[178]

'And it's not the Danny Frawleys in their fifties or the Polly Farmers in their eighties,' he continues. 'We're talking about guys in their early twenties who have said, "I'd like to retire because I have too many concussions and I can't work or I can't even work for three hours before my brain shuts down. I can't even exercise. I haven't walked out of the house for two years because I can't handle the noise or the light or too many people," or someone else goes, "Well, I can't go to the shop because I get completely overwhelmed."'[179]

There's AFL player Justin Clarke who played for the Brisbane Lions, and was forced to retire from the AFL in 2016 at 22 years old after an incident at training left him seriously concussed, which affected his memory and mobility.[180] And Melbourne defender Kade Kolodjashnij who announced in 2020 that he was taking early AFL retirement due to a concussion.

'The writing was on the wall ever since that knock 12 months ago, that I knew my time might be up and that my body just couldn't keep up with the demands of AFL,' he said in the *Herald Sun*. 'Doctors have said to me that it's probably best I finish up for health reasons.'

In April 2021, Pearce released results from the Australian Sports Brain Bank that found more than 80 per cent of the 162 retired VFL/AFL players he had tested were suffering from a form of brain damage, with the remaining players showing some abnormalities when compared to age-matched healthy controls, suggesting that their experiences in playing had affected their brains.

The latest from Australia is a world-first study of league players that finds no link between concussions and depression risk, co-authored by neuropsychologist Andrew Gardner, an associate professor at the University of Newcastle's School of Medicine and Public Health.

The paper hypothesised that if athletes had been reading a lot of things that have been reported from North America through the media or are looking at the narrative that is typically 'If you have concussions, you're going to have all of these difficulties', then, in the co-authors' words, 'it becomes a self-fulfilling prophecy ... Once you start reading all of that you become hypervigilant,' he says, 'so you leave your keys behind or lose your mobile phone – everyone does that – but you think you have memory problems. The difficulty has been that the narrative has been monopolised by one group in North America, and it's always been really negative.'[181]

I have yet to find a positive spin on concussion.

'I can't play the whole "concussions are a concern but we shouldn't be concerned about long-term issues as its all sensationalised" line', Pearce agrees. 'I have both young and old athletes, elite and non-elite, males and now a growing number of females, sometimes emotionally broken by these neurologists saying that it will all just resolve and take time,' he says. 'But it hasn't.'

'Remember that politics, colonialism, imperialism and war also originate in the human brain.'
— Vilayanur S. Ramachandran, neuroscientist

Chapter Six

A Culture of Pain

I find Kat on social media. In 2018, Kat tweeted about her husband Chris's concussions — that's actually how I found her. Chris Czekaj has now retired from playing professional rugby for Wales.

'He still has plans to be a player coach of a local rugby team. He's coaching at the moment,' she tells me. 'If I had my way, he'd be probably hanging his boots up. I can't really tell him what to do!' She laughs, but there is an underlying note of concern in her tone.

On the whole, Kat is animated, taking me through the beginning of her and Chris's relationship. They met while he was playing for the Cardiff RFC, in 2005, and they've been together for 16 years.

'He was slender back then, used to be so quick. In fact, he was brilliant. He was like lightning on the pitch!' she says, sounding still in awe, I think.

In the first seven months of their relationship, Chris went from playing semi-professionally with the Cardiff RFC to getting called up for the Welsh squad. He was training full time, with one match day a week. Chris grabbed the opportunity with both hands, Kat says. He thrived in the team.

'He went for very long periods without even a nick,' she says to me. 'He played every game and was fit and healthy for the entire time. And then he broke his leg playing for Wales against Australia [in 2007] and it went downhill from there.'[182]

Chris had broken his femur in five different places. It splintered and fragmented into six separate parts. During the operation the surgeon told Kat that he had only ever seen this kind of injury in motorcycle crashes.

It was serious, but all Chris wanted to know was when he would be able to play rugby again, to which the doctor responded: 'I want to get you to a point where you are able to walk again and play in the park with your children.'

Kat says that over the next 18 months, Chris displayed the most intense mental resolve she had ever seen. He put absolutely everything into his rehabilitation; his focus on getting back in the game was powering him through. At the end of that time, he was back on the pitch having signed on to the Cardiff Blues: he'd gone full circle, back to where he started.

'And from that point I didn't actually watch any of the rugby that was happening, I was just constantly focused on what he was doing, where he was on the pitch. I watched it very differently from that moment on,' Kat admits.

She became a lot more protective of him – matches became harder to watch. She certainly didn't enjoy watching him play anymore. There were other injuries during that time back at the Cardiff Blues. He had quite a few concussions, Kat tells me, maybe three, or four. Definitely three serious ones and a couple of other bumps.

'But on the pitch, they'd just be like, are you OK? This was in 2009 before HIAs [Head Injury Assessments] were fully written into rugby law.'

There is no suggestion from Kat that the medical team at the time were incompetent, but rather they just operated under different guidelines back then. She is certain that if it was now, they would have noted all of the areas of concern and taken him off. But at this time, in his own words, he took a 'bang to the head' against Gloucester, and just played on.

'He actually can't remember any of the second half,' Kat says. 'I think this highlights that you don't have to be knocked out to be concussed, which is a common misconception – even just a bang to the head will do it.'

I can't hide my surprise that they allowed him to play on. 'But the worst one was when we were living in France,' she adds quickly, as if the Gloucester match was a mere aside. 'That match in France was the worst day of my life. It really was.'

On 11 April 2014, the Cardiff Blues announced that Czekaj would be joining France's Pro D2 rugby team, US Colomiers, at the end of the 2013/14 season. The family were all there to watch his first match. Chris had gone up for a high ball but came off the wrong end of it, taking a hit to his head.

'I saw him go up and then I saw players screaming for medical staff,' Kat says. 'And I'm looking at all the players still standing, thinking, *Where's Christopher?* Then, *Oh, my God, no.*'[183]

She saw the players become frantic. The crowd had gone silent.

'I stood up and ran down the steps because I suddenly realised, you know, I think that's Christopher. And I could just see him on the floor fitting and having this huge convulsion. He was purple. You don't know what to think at that point.'

Kat had grabbed her son, who was just over two at the time, and ran around the side of the pitch to the tunnel.

'I didn't really speak much French but I'm there screaming, "Help me, let me in!" ' They let her into the tunnel just as Chris was wheeled past. 'They had actually intubated him because he had stopped breathing.'

They took Chris into the medical room but wouldn't let Kat come in. She waited outside for 20 minutes, banging on the door, begging to be beside him. The answer was no, there were people rushing around that needed space, you need to stay out there.

'And I'm thinking, *My God, he's dead here,*' Kat says. 'Like, here I am, I'm holding my son . . . I'm frantic, I'm watching all these people. And I just don't know what to think!'

Her words remind me of Karen in the hospital, trying to find her son, Benjamin. Another rugby-related injury. An awful outcome.

'It was the longest 20 minutes and then eventually the doctor came up to me, said, "Oh, he's OK. He's come to. We'll let you in in a minute." '

We both release the breaths neither of us realise we've been holding. 'So, they took me into the room and Chris sat up and he's like, "Oh, hello, are you OK?" '

It was as if nothing had happened; instead the doctor tried to lighten the mood by showing her where Chris's jaw had clamped down on his hand after he'd wrenched his mouth open in fear of him swallowing his gumshield – or worse, his tongue.

A hospital trip followed, with a diagnosis of the highest grade of concussion. Kat was told they could go home but to keep an eye on him for the next week or so. She reiterates that the period between the match and the hospital was awful but that what followed was even more disturbing.

Chris had huge black eyes that were bloodshot, he was drained and physically tired to the point where he didn't seem like he was there at all.

'I watched him change pretty much overnight,' she says. 'He was physically present, but his mind was just . . .' She searches for the words. 'Like, he was looking at you, but he was just seeing straight through you,' she finishes, much quieter now.

Chris, who Kat describes as the most chilled person she had ever met in her life – the guy who was fazed by nothing, the guy who never raised his voice – became aggressive. He had no patience: he became angry at the smallest things and was sleeping a lot. Kat recalls Chris leaving the room at one point, letting her know he'd be back in a second, only he never returned.

Concerned, Kat walked around the house only to find him in the bedroom standing in front of the curtains, very close to the fabric. 'He looked like he was in a different world and he said, "I don't know where the bathroom is."' They'd been living in their house for three months at this point. Chris doesn't remember any of this happening.

'But ever since then, I've noticed differences in his personality and the intricacies of, you know, who he is. That has slightly changed. He's not as patient as he was at all. I think he does wonder what the future might be like. And that scares me a lot. It's not just a bump on the head, like people say,' she says, referring to concussion.

Kat makes a good point. I've been thinking a lot about the integral role that language plays in brain injury, on so many levels.

Terms like 'head knocks', which were still being used in 2021[184] and downplay the severity of a concussion. Which is dangerous not only to other peer professionals but also to aspiring amateur players. Nobody wants to appear weak in sport, especially one where defiance and strength are the key components.

A lot of players have openly admitted to holding their shoulders as they're walking off a field, trying to hide the symptomology and not acknowledge to the cameras or even to a physio that they had a head injury. From a professional point of view, a head injury will have an impact on how frequently they play, their future contracts, their involvement with the team and the games in the weeks that follow. The culture that exists means that even if players have some knowledge of the severity of their situation, they may feel the need to disguise it. How much is this driven by the expectations of the coaches, big bosses, leagues? The feeling of not wanting to let their teammates, families or fans down? How much is it the fear that someone else is waiting on the sidelines, ready to take their place?

Ed Daly, a former rugby coach and researcher, tells me of a match a couple of years ago in the All-Ireland League, a top division of Irish rugby, where a player, clearly concussed, was refusing to go off. He started sobbing with his face in the mud, the concussion triggering a massive emotional response that left him crying and shuddering. 'I don't want to go off,' he was repeating, yet he was quite visibly concussed. It reminded me of Peter Robinson saying that sports eat protocol, and the players exist in a culture of 'get up and get on with it, stop moaning'.[185]

While studies have proved that the awareness and the knowledge around concussion is high, with education and conversations increasing across the globe, what isn't changing is the culture. There is still a growing emphasis on being bigger, especially in rugby, even at schoolboy age: that the bigger the player,

the bigger the tackles. You only have to look at the size of the
Saracens' players, the English professional rugby team based in
London – a team built on massive guys that other people just
can't compete with, and who sustain really large hits as a result.
There is an aggression attached to teams of their size that per-
petuates a testosterone-driven atmosphere. If you're big, strong
and aggressive then it follows that surely you should be able to
take the blows? And, if you want to do well, really well, you stay
on the pitch, no matter what.

★★★

I'm standing in another kitchen staring at another dining table
covered in piles of documents, cease and desist letters, photographs and newspaper articles similar to those I've seen at
Dawn Astle's. They belong to Sam Peters, an award-winning
former sports journalist and media campaigner.

'We're about to move out of town to the countryside,' he
says by way of explanation, catching my gaze; but it's not the
volume of documents that has my attention, it's the fact that
he's kept them for so long. It was Dawn herself that suggested
I contact him. He tells me I've found him at a good time. He's
got a lot to say because frankly, he says, he's pissed off with what
he regards as sport 'failing to act when there were opportunities
to act and failing to act when more evidence emerged.' He says,
'And that's not even just failing to act, but actually construc-
tively making the situation worse by choosing to play more
games in a week!'[186]

I ask the RFU how they are reacting to the evidence
that is emerging; it's a stock response as expected that reads
'Through many years of research and monitoring we now

144

have far more data, which has allowed us to improve concussion surveillance, education and management as well as all injury prevention and injury treatment.' They go on to say that 'While rugby is a contact sport, the care and focus on concussion education, recognition and management for players is the best that it has ever been, and we will continue to use the latest evidence and research to keep improving.' They then direct me to HEADCASE, Rugby's concussion awareness and education materials, which were developed in 2013 in consultation with Headway and leading neurologists and are now 'recognised as the leading concussion awareness and education materials in the UK'.

'The campaign comprises two simple messages: "the four Rs (recognise, remove, recover, return)" and "if in doubt, sit them out".'

I know those words: it's what Peter Robinson uses to advocate for Benjamin.

Sam Peters has a lot more to say. He is friendly and well spoken. He speaks quickly, with an enthusiasm for each of the words he chooses. He is a former rugby player and an avid fan of the sport. It was this passion that led him into sports journalism and ultimately to become a seminal figure in the discussion on brain injury in sport. He spearheaded the *Mail on Sunday*'s 'Concussion in Rugby' campaign back in 2013, although he has an almost knee-jerk reaction to bat away any praise.

'I think I could just see the wood for the trees,' Sam says. 'You know, just maybe I was a bit closer to some of the players because of my age profile. I left school in '96, started to play Union in '97. I spent a year in the army between school and university, played rugby all the way through from school, through uni, and knew a lot of guys who'd go on to play professionally.'

Sam was getting a lot of information out of some of the dressing rooms, which he thinks others probably weren't hearing, especially in the early days of the professional game.

Having reported on the game for decades, he realised that since the year Rugby Union went professional, in 1995, the game had grown exponentially, most noticeably in the physique of the players. A former player I spoke with likened the rapid advance to the Fat Boy Slim music video for 'Right Here, Right Now', which depicts man's evolution across 4.2 billion years in just four and a half minutes.[187] Now the athletes are bigger, stronger, they play with less fear and more ferocity; there is more muscle, more power, and they are in training several times a week ahead of matches. There are also more matches.

Sam felt that along with the increase in the players' size and the ferocity of play, that concussions had become much more prevalent, and while he admits there were a lot of benefits – quite a lot of 'associated glory, for want of a better expression' – he acknowledges that also a 'heck of a lot of negatives just weren't being spoken about'.[188]

Sam knew first-hand how violent the game could be, having suffered from three rugby injuries, leading to surgery and several concussions. He knew what it was like to sit in a hospital bed waiting for the surgeon to come round with an anaesthetist to knock him out, not knowing what you could wake up with afterwards.

He was concerned that players were being put at extreme risk.

'I didn't really understand what that actually meant,' Sam says. 'I didn't really think there was any science to back up my concern or any kind of interest in the story, but as the NFL story began to sort of grow and we began to understand more and more, I started to wonder, well, what's the difference between the NFL and rugby?'

These are big guys hitting very, very hard and relentlessly over long periods of time, he thought. So, why is a head injury different in rugby to American football to boxing to a car accident? The more people he spoke to, the more he realised that there could be a problem that no one was admitting.

'I was kind of a persona non grata for quite a long time,' he laughs, but it gave him the confidence to investigate further. What did they have to hide? 'The very people who were most annoyed by what I was doing were exactly the people I wanted to be annoyed by it,' he says simply.

In 2013, a headline in the *Mail on Sunday* read that rugby was a ticking time bomb.[189] The article by Sam Peters and Daniel Schofield linked brain damage and dementia among players to the increasing number of head injuries. It cited examples of injured players and experts who believed that the current concussion protocol was 'dangerous'. Chris Nowinski said: 'There is evidence of a concussion problem in rugby similar to that in the NFL. It is not just an American football problem . . . When you engage in something that involves repeated brain trauma with force, it opens the door to serious problems.'[190] Dr Willie Stewart is quoted as saying, 'If we liken this to a marathon, then the gun has only just gone off [...] It would be foolish to think rugby is immune to brain damage.' Dr Willie Stewart was one of the experts quoted in Peters and Schofield's 2013 article. A consultant neuropathologist who has played a pivotal role in the UK's concussion and CTE research over the last 20 years, he released clinical research of what he believed to be the first confirmed case of early onset dementia caused by playing rugby. Like Peters, Dr Stewart was a former player and avid fan himself and had become increasingly concerned at what he was seeing when watching matches.

The RFU head of sports medicine, Dr Simon Kemp, is quoted in the article as saying 'that the union were committed to delivering best practice in the handling of concussion cases'. But he also said: 'We understand that there is no proven causal relationship between head injuries sustained while playing rugby union and the reported cases of CTE and early-onset dementia.'

On the surface of things after the article, changes were made very quickly. The RFU implemented compulsory education programmes for players, coaches and referees and pretty much everyone associated with the professional game. They also introduced a head injury assessment, called the Pitch Side Concussion Assessment (PCSA), which had initially been a five-minute test on the side of the pitch and was later changed to ten minutes. In the 1980s, if you were suspected of having a concussion, the mandatory stand down period was three weeks.

And yet we're now at a point where the game has evolved so much since it was professionalised in the 1990s that it is almost unrecognisable in terms of both the physicality of the players who have now been deemed 'colossal'[191] and of the sport itself. The more powerful the players, the greater the ramifications of the impacts during play.[192] There is a greater force being exerted on the guys' heads in every single match. Often in the slow-motion action replays you can visibly see the heads of players whipping back, their features seeming to slide off the side of their face with the sheer impact.

'I would now argue that rugby's gone beyond the NFL in terms of that,' Peters says. 'In fact, it's way beyond the NFL in terms of the physical demands, because, and anyone in the NFL would laugh at that, but the amount of contacts that, say, a flanker in rugby is asked to take every single game, if we carry every tackle, every breakdown, every one of those is a subconcussive scenario and every one of those is a risk of a concussive episode happening.'[193]

★★★

'I've said for several years now that from what we know about American football and boxing there is absolutely no reason at all to expect rugby is immune from this disease unless they are saying that people who play rugby have a completely different brain to the rest of us,' he said in the article.[194]

If you look at the data across different sports, a footballer is three and a half times more likely to develop a degenerative brain disease than the global population.[195] The American football mortality data is pretty much the same; despite the sport being incredibly high impact, players are only on the pitch for a few minutes at a time in a match. Therefore, the higher impact of the sport is matched by less time on the pitch, carrying a similar risk to UK football.

'But then you put rugby in the mix, which is an 80-minute game with remarkable rates of impact during the week in training and phenomenal amounts of injury on match days in professional rugby,' Dr Stewart says. So much so that rugby is now recording one brain injury per match consistently for several years now.[196] 'That, to me, is both remarkable and unacceptable that the game is continuing to see this happen,' he adds.

I agree that one player being taken off the pitch per match with a suspected mild brain injury is astonishing, especially as there is a risk that these injuries may be more serious. Acute brain injury issues can often follow, though sports have made an effort to increase the return-to-play time to ensure a recovery is made. Back in the 1990s this was 21 days as standard, although some players have returned within 24 hours. The dialogue around an appropriate length of time has long been debated, with sporting bodies finally seeming to be listening and making adjustments, yet it seems to me that longer-term degeneration is still being ignored.

'There's no question that this will feed into issues to do with the degenerative brain disease as well,' Dr Stewart says, 'because what we are seeing are rugby players from the so-called amateur era, players from the '50s and '60s and later, and we are seeing chronic traumatic encephalopathy pathology in their brains. Essentially, we're seeing the same pathologies you see in footballers and American football players. And that's from the amateur era.'[197]

There is something else that coincides with the mis-communication surrounding injury, which is a common misunderstanding about the human brain itself. That it is unbreakable, strong enough to withstand trauma because of its casing within the skull and that a helmet protects the brain, creating a false sense of security for both the players and the spectators. Putting on 'armour' always feels safer, placing a barrier between what needs to be protected and what can cause harm. It seems rational, doesn't it? But a helmet will only protect the player from abrasions, cuts and fractures; it also keeps the skull together if it cracks. The brain tissue itself is extremely soft and extremely delicate. Helmets do not protect the brain against concussion. That is caused when the brain is rattled inside the skull; helmets do next to nothing to prevent that.

To put it in context, the brain is much softer than a piece of raw meat that you might buy in the supermarket. If you think about squeezing a piece of raw meat between your fingers and compressing it, then it is easy to flatten out and squash down. So, when a force is applied to the head, the brain is actually being compressed and stretched and twisted and when a force comes in on one side, the brain is essentially sloshed over to the other side and pressed up against the inside of the skull. It deforms considerably.

I'm not sure we really appreciate how much the brain is being physically changed as a result of these relatively modest impacts. We've come to equate the brain with being powerful, similar to the smart phones we all have, neurons in our pockets made of sturdy gorilla glass, supposedly unbreakable, engineered to protect against damage. But the brain is undoubtedly the most fragile organ in our body.

In addition to the deformity, the essential level of where the injury is at in the brain is increasingly recognised to be in what we call the white matter of the brain.

So, while the brain is a soft, squishy kilo-and-a-half piece of tissue, it is composed of hundreds of billions of cells. These cells are unique in that they are all connected to each other by a very fine network, a web that is more complex than the internet. These connections are extremely delicate, which means that the impact of the deformity places a remarkable amount of stress on that network.

Stress in the form of stretching and twisting of these axons is going to lead to changes in their microscopic structure and function, which the body has a tremendous ability to repair; the brain is incredibly resilient to injury because even things that we do all the time, like running and jumping, can cause deformity in this way.

But it is the repetition of these impacts over time that can overwhelm the repair mechanisms, which can cause an injury to develop. Inflammation can also occur in the brain as a response to the injury, which in itself can cause further damage. It's a vicious cycle and I wonder why it isn't taken as seriously as, say, a broken leg.

If we break a leg, we rest it immediately, we take our weight off it. Later, it will be encased in plaster, protected. Perhaps, the brain feels too conceptual: broken bones are tangible, the mind and the brain are not, not really. Once a bone is broken, it's broken, and we can physically see that on an X-ray; we can pinpoint exactly where the damage is and therefore determine its severity. Ultimately, we know what we're dealing with; there is no grey area. But trauma to the brain is like a bruise on a bruise on a bruise, only we just can't see it.

Maybe as humans we need that immediate feedback in order to acknowledge what is happening – nothing screams 'time out' like the crack of a bone or a fountain of blood or the searing pain of a snapped tendon. It's as if blood and broken bones are an emphasis of how strong you went or played: you went so hard that you cracked a bone, *what a warrior*.

I can't help but wonder if brain injury sits within the realm of 'softness', like mindfulness does for so many. It's been called a conspiracy even in supposedly 'woke' news outlets. Any negative discourse is usually accompanied by effeminate language seeming to diminish its integrity. It's here I can see the remnants of Muscular Christians the most. I can see how this could transpire on the pitch – if you're the star player and you're going to go off mid-game, you'd better have a good reason. Crowds and stadiums have clapped and cheered for their fallen hero's broken bones and bloodied noses as marks of accomplishment, a visual indication that a player has gone above and beyond, that they've made the sacrifice for the greater good. Because if a player is seen to falter, then not only does he face the wrath of the stadium, but also his team-mates, coaches, transfers and ultimately contracts – everything is at stake.

'The money goes both ways,' Dr Willie Stewart tells me. 'Sport needs the attention of participation to generate income. Let's not pretend that the global game of football is there so we can see people kick a ball around. It's a global entertainment industry out to make money. But on the other hand, you know, people in research are also desperate to generate income as well. Otherwise, they can't do the research. So, there's money on both sides, though there's a lot more money in the entertainment industry than in the research.'[198]

He suggests that there are those that may have a vested interest in there not being a connection between repetitive head injury and later-life issues, and there are those who are connected to tertiary institutions where they are perhaps encouraged not to be part of controversy. Then there are those who have been accused of deliberately failing to warn players about the dangers of their sport, when their role is to protect them.

Following McKee's CTE diagnosis, Aaron Hernandez's attorneys filed a lawsuit against the NFL and the New England Patriots in U.S. district court on behalf of Hernandez's four-year-old daughter, Avielle, seeking financial damages for the loss of her father.[199]

NFL spokesman Joe Lockhart told reporters that the NFL intended to 'vigorously' contest the lawsuit, saying it would face 'significant legal issues from the start'.[200] That lawsuit was subsequently dropped and a new lawsuit was filed in Norfolk County Superior Court against the NFL and helmet maker Riddell.

Riddell was the NFL's helmet maker from 1989 to 2014. In 2002 they had begun to develop and market a new helmet designed to reduce players' risk of concussions. It would go on to become the most widely used helmet in the NFL. Bought by millions. It was named 'The Revolution'.[201]

In 2000 an Ottawa-based biomechanical firm, which was also working with the NFL's Minor Traumatic Brain Injury (MTBI) Committee to study head injuries and test the helmets, had sent a report to Riddell that stated that there was a 'high frequency of concussion in the game of football, despite the quality of today's headgear'.[202] The report suggested that the helmets and the safety tests used to regulate them were designed to prevent catastrophic head injuries like skull fractures, but little research had been previously conducted when it came to preventing concussions.

Despite this, the brand became the most popular helmet in the NFL, with 84 per cent of players wearing them in 2008.[203]

That report was referred to in a 2013 Colorado lawsuit,[204] in which Riddell was found liable for $3.1 million out of a total of $11.5 million that was awarded to the family of a former football player who was seriously injured after a concussion in a high-school football practice. The Colorado jury cleared Riddell of the charge that its helmet had a design flaw. But it found that the company had failed to adequately warn players of the risks of potential concussions. In a statement Riddell said they were pleased that 'the jury determined that Riddell's helmet was not defective in any way' but that they intended to appeal this verdict, stating 'we remain steadfast in our belief that Riddell designs and manufactures the most protective football headgear for the athlete'.

The company have since faced a number of lawsuits, including one brought forth in Ohio by the family of a 22-year-old, who suffered a seizure while fishing and drowned. Coby Hamblin died in 2016, five years after he stopped playing football.

His family claim the seizure was a result of brain damage he had suffered during his ten years of play.

Following a post-mortem, it was discovered that Hamblin had Stage II CTE.

A judge ruled that five of the six claims against Riddell by Hamblin's father would be allowed to proceed including wrongful death, strict liability for design defect, strict liability for manufacturing defect, defects in warning or instructions and defect by failure to conform to representation.

In a statement Ridell said, 'Plaintiff's allegations are unproven and vigorously contested. The Court's ruling dismissed plaintiff's fraud claim while simply allowing others to proceed past this very initial pleadings stage (...) The plaintiff's allegations face many other challenges before they could ever reach a trial, and Riddell is confident in its defense to these meritless claims.'

The lawsuit is ongoing.

It was ultimately ruled by a federal judge that Avielle Hernandez could not sue the NFL over CTE. The lawsuit against the NFL was dismissed, but Riddell was not addressed in that judgement, according to the official order of dismissal from judge Anita B. Brody: 'A.H. also names Riddell Inc., the manufacturer of the helmets worn by NFL football players, and related entities as defendants. Because only the NFL Parties have moved to dismiss A.H.'s claims, I will not address A.H.'s claims against the Riddell Defendants.'[205]

The 2017 claim was moved to Federal court, where it was also dismissed.

The judge did not acknowledge Riddell in the ruling.

In a 2017 statement emailed to the Associated Press, Riddell said such legal action 'harms the game of football and the many millions of participants whose lives have been enriched' by sports. It continued, 'This latest copycat complaint, like the ones preceding it, demonstrates little regard for the implications that sensationalized allegations have on the sport and the millions of people who benefit from it.'[206]

But what is clear from the 'The Revolution' is that language is a defining factor in the interrogation of CTE and determines how seriously brain injury is taken by athletes, the public and sport itself.

This is often perpetuated by the media and certainly experts in the field who present predominantly sports-friendly viewpoints, which minimise the risks of concussion and head injuries, while simultaneously downplaying connections between sport and neurodegenerative disease, meaning it doesn't fall under a 'serious injury' category.

In 2017, Irish football manager and former player Roy Keane was quoted as saying in a press conference:'If you're worried about the physical side of any sport then play chess. [...] It's part of the game. Whether it be hurling, football, American football or rugby . .. People question the PFA, but when you cross that line there's an element of risk involved, a chance you might get hurt.'[207]

In *The Matrix: An Exploration of the Interactions between the Economy, War, and Economic Theory*, Michael Perelman and Vincent Portillo link the authoritarian nature of coaching to that of business management.[208] They assert that where sport resonated with the grander cultural aspirations of the leaders of American universities, who accepted the ideals of Muscular Christianity as a means of developing character, they also must have appreciated that football games earned them good revenues.

Scoring points as a team has been said to resemble the way corporations kept the books on profits, which flowed from the collective efforts of their workers. Time management was a crucial consideration in running a business as well as a football game. Knowing when to slow down, knowing when to up the pace, knowing how to use those fundamental few seconds before the final whistle blows, that can be the difference between victory and despair, to your advantage. Or rather, to the advantage of your club, whatever it costs.

And while sporting heroes are cherished and adored, they are never really protected or secure like those in power. The gladiators were generally former slaves or prisoners, and while they could rise to fame, they were never truly unchained, only owned and traded among masters like prized assets.

Dylan Hartley, the former England rugby captain and author of *The Hurt*, uses the phrase 'industrialised brutality' in the first chapter of his memoir, which is aptly titled 'Meat', stating that 'rugby is great for the soul, but terrible for the body'.[209] He goes on to say, 'I eventually became sick of living on painkillers, of having my life controlled by aspirations to play for England.'

'You know churn rate, if that was for want of a better enumeration, we shouldn't ever use that to describe human beings,' Sam Peters says. 'If you're talking about assets and damaging assets, it's like sport's most prized assets are being damaged on a routine basis. What other business does that? To its best assets? Shouldn't we protect them instead of breaking them before they've reached their peak? It's utterly crazy.'

Yet sport still remains aspirational.

'Kids don't know the danger,' Sam says. 'And if they do it's from their parents. But when you're on a field, you're still going to do it because you like playing. You don't want to sit on a bench.'

In reality though, as with the AFL, rugby is now seeing younger men, in their late twenties to mid-thirties – not their fifties and sixties – describing the pain their bodies have been put through, including the high-profile players, such as James Haskell, Sam Burgess and former England captain Hartley – who Sam Peters described as 'one of the toughest men on the planet'.

Sam lists Jack Clifford, who recently retired at 27 years old, and should have, in Sam's opinion, had 70 England caps ahead of him. We go a little further back to Tom Reese who should have had 70 caps too, but retired at 26 years old.

Sam Peters still loves the game, even though he can't play anymore due to injury. 'I still look back now, and I love it. But once you get to the point of being professional, everything changes in terms of the relationship between you and your club ... It becomes a professional commercial arrangement and your employer should have a duty of care. Instead, it's like [the players are] being thought of as commodities.'

I also put this to the RFU directly, that players were being used as commodities and were considered disposable. They stated that 'The RFU takes player safety very seriously and implements concussion and all injury prevention and treatment strategies based on the latest research and evidence.'

But it didn't really address the why. Why the players were retiring so young if it was being taken very seriously. Why is the former England captain absolutely destroyed in mind and body if the game is safe?

Appearing as a co-host on an episode of the *RugbyPass Offload* podcast, ex-England captain Hartley said that he didn't know dementia could be a potential outcome for any rugby player. 'That wasn't educated or taught to us,' he said. 'It's scary to think that NFL has had CTE and issues with this injury for some time and we play a very similar sport and we have never recognised it in our players.'[210]

'The thrill of victory . . . and the agony of defeat.'[211]
— Jim McKay, sports commentator

Chapter Seven

The Tip of the Iceberg

My fascination with sport began early on. I went through a phase as a child of secretly wanting to be a football commentator when I grew up. We would listen to matches on the radio in my dad's car. I loved the excited crescendo of their voices, elongating their words for dramatic effect and *speeeeeeedingupeverytimeaplayerwasneara- GOAAAAAAAAL!*

It was thrilling, even just to listen to, and I thought it sounded like the best job in the world. I enjoyed watching sport much more than playing it. I was a small, skinny, artsy child with allergies who paled in comparison to the strength of the farming-family offspring at my village school, with their broad shoulders and lineage of plough-pulling strength. But I loved the energy of a crowd, the buzz of a stadium, the performance of it all; how it transcended sport itself into something much more visceral – the artistry, the dedication, the celebration. You could get lost in a good match like a good plot in a movie. I liked when it kept you on your toes, the promise that anything could happen – even a miracle, especially a miracle.

It was the fans' devotion to sport that fascinated me the most. I was stunned by its power. I had seen it take hold of those I knew on numerous occasions; witnessed their tears of joy and pain on account of 11 or 15 of 'their' men lifting or not lifting a trophy as though the world, or at least *their* world, depended on it. I had been privy to both the kissing of strangers' faces in bars that followed the former, and the three-day sulks and the 'I-just-can't-talk-about-it-yet's that followed the latter. Later, I found that sport was able to draw out emotions that I had long given up on eliciting in hardened, self-proclaimed 'closed-book' men, bursting their pages and tear ducts open effortlessly. It brought adults to their knees, on and off the pitch, regardless of class, country or language. Sport was inclusive, sure, but above all, sport was sacred.

In September 2008, in an article titled 'The Cult of Football: A Religion for the Twentieth Century and Beyond', Illya McLellan describes sport as 'a religion that would in some ways inspire more devotion and fervour than its tired counterparts that were still mired in the doctrines of yesteryear'.[212]

There are many comparisons to be drawn between sport and religious iconography, too. The kneeling in celebration of a goal, that split-second action, offering oneself up to the 'gods', be it metaphorically or literally, to the highest row of seats at the back of the stadium, that declares 'I am here to serve you'. Even the language used in sport discussion has a religious undertone; cult phrases like 'a hail Mary', 'the hand of god' or commentators describing stadiums as 'a screaming hell' or the 'trance-like' chorus from the fans. Religion focuses on the idea that there is something more to the world than meets the eye. That 'something' is the domain of the divine; in sport, that 'something' is the triumph of the human spirit.

We are reminded of this from time to time, when we witness the rise of a supremely gifted athlete who simultaneously takes our breath away and affirms our hope that the impossible just might actually be possible. We crave a champion, a working-class hero to rise like a phoenix from the ashes of circumstance and take the world stage. No one exemplifies this better than the Argentine, Diego Maradona. Following Argentina's World Cup win in 1968, sports journalist Daniel Arcucci described the country's reaction to Maradona as 'celebrating its saviour'.

In news footage following his first match for Napoli in 1984, Maradona himself is seen crediting God first and foremost for his ability, for allowing him a goal, despite the match being lost. The Neapolitans shower him with adoration; here he is, the answer to their prayers in human form. As Napoli climb the league table, ultimately the adoration intensifies. In Maradona, they not only have a gifted athlete, a defiant figure, but the hope for something better. Nothing has the ability to bring a society together quite like sports can. A nurse even left a vial of Maradona's blood on a shrine in a Catholic church as if he were a god. When Napoli wins its first title, a banner is hung along a wall at the entrance to a cemetery, a message to the dead: 'You don't know what you missed.'

I had another taste of this, watching the 2018 World Cup when, for the first time in years, the whole of the UK was united in its optimism that football might actually be coming home, courtesy of Gareth Southgate's England Team. It happened again in 2021, during the Euros, when emerging from the tragedy of a pandemic, we finally had something to believe in. We followed their trials with great devotion; we had the utmost faith in our team and its captain and worshipped their efforts. And if that's not an ideology, then what is?

It all changed in the final on 11 July 2021 when England failed to bring home the trophy, losing to Italy in penalties. Adoration quickly turned to devastation, which escalated to rage. Players that had been heralded for weeks, Marcus Rashford, Jadon Sancho and Bukayo Saka were racially abused on social media for missing their penalties and a mural celebrating Rashford in Manchester was defaced overnight.

I think back to Maradona, to the power he held, but how quickly 'God' became 'the Devil', or 'Lucifer', to quote the Italian media after the controversial 1990 World Cup semi-final that saw Argentina, Maradona's home country, beat Italy at home in Napoli, his club at the time.

Maradona was never in charge of his own fate, he belonged to the people and to his club. This is best exemplified when he pleaded for a transfer that was refused by the Napoli President Corrado Ferlaino, who said, on reflection, 'I was Maradona's jailer.'[213]

Although we build up the players to almost immortal status, I have to question who really calls the shots – not who was playing God as such – but who has the power to make decisions, not just regarding the fate of a team, but an individual's life, like Maradona's, too?

***

At a test match at London's Lord's Cricket Ground, during a discussion on the campaign, a friend of journalist Sam Peters, Jim Holden, said that he should speak to Dawn Astle.

Sam remembered Jeff Astle from *Fantasy Football*. He knew he'd been a very good player and had a vague recollection of reading about the neurological problems he'd encountered subsequent to playing.

'I guess like many people reading at the time that there was gonna be a big PFA–FA-led inquiry into the potential risk of head injuries in football, I wrongly assumed that that had been carried out . . . obviously they hadn't found anything and therefore, you know, nothing to see here, no problem,' Peters says.

Jim Holden had done a bit of looking around himself, online, in newspapers, but the biggest research project ever funded by the FA and PFA to look into industrial disease linked to hitting footballs or head injuries in football, which had caused Jeff's death, was nowhere to be found.

'And so, the more questions I asked,' Sam says, 'and the more I looked into it, the more I became convinced that the study had never actually happened. There was nothing online, no one had the same story, nothing joined up and the only conclusion I could draw was that it basically had been kicked into the long grass and hadn't been properly carried out, and obviously I then stopped to think, *Well, what are the consequences of this?*'[214]

He didn't know then that those consequences would forever alter the course of the Astles' lives, and that of many others who followed. At the time it was just a story Sam Peters decided was definitely worth printing. He felt there were two people that he needed to speak to before he went ahead and published it though: Dawn and Laraine Astle.

'And then, well, it turned into Pandora's Box,' Sam Peters says with the hint of a smile.

Yes, I think, this is a story that had initially felt like a gift but with the potential to turn into a curse, bringing with it great and unexpected troubles. I still feel that now. But trouble for who? Who's being protected if the lid's left on?

'It's one I'm prepared to open,' I say to Sam. His smile widens.

***

The Astles had been waiting for the ten-year joint study that the PFA and FA had jointly launched before Jeff's death to investigate any possible link between heading footballs and an increased prevalence of neurodegenerative illnesses among ex-professional players.[215]

'They . . . they promised,' Laraine Astle says, holding the last word in her mouth for a moment, her tongue almost rejecting the syllables. 'They promised,' she repeats, her tone firmer now. 'So, we thought the research was ongoing [and] nobody really could say how long it was going to go on for.'[216]

Twelve years after Jeff's death, Laraine Astle received a phone call from Sam Peters, a journalist working for the *Mail on Sunday*. 'And he said, ever so polite he was, "Oh, Mrs Astle, I understand the FA are doing this study, can I come and see you?"'

Laraine knew to call her daughters whenever a journalist was enquiring about their dad; it was something she had become used to. By the time Dawn arrived at Laraine's house, Sam Peters was already there sitting on a chair.

My eyes flit around Laraine's living room once more, the images of Jeff, the England caps, a space that has seen so much joy and suffering within its four walls, where residues of memory sit like dormant dust, ready to be swirled up again with every visiting guest that has come to ask questions, myself included.

Maybe it gets easier each time, I think, to settle the thoughts back down once they've been disturbed again. But there is something about the vividness of Laraine and Dawn's recollections that suggest another two decades could pass and the pain would still be just as palpable. It's then that the reality of this unique situation hurtles into focus. Are we helping? Are we making it worse?

If I catch myself before my ego's defences are in place, I feel guilty asking people to walk me through their pain. I remember hearing a war zone photographer detail the moment he had taken an image of a child dying on the backseat of a car in a conflict zone, the child's eyes were open, and the photographer realised he could see the reflection of his camera lens in her pupils, the reflection as sharp as glass. It hit him then that the last thing this child would see would be his camera pointing in her face, not his hand outstretched to help her, as if the realisation of what he was doing suddenly pulled into focus for the very first time, despite years in the field. It opens up an interesting discussion on the exploitation of tragedy. Is it OK if we are telling the truth? If we are showing the world for what it is?

The title of 'journalist' or 'photo-journalist' facilitates this idea that we are allowed to step a little closer, that certain rules don't apply, that we are allowed to ask harder questions. It's a strange dichotomy – it's never about me, and yet being the one to tell the truth is wrapped up in the singularity – that I am the 'one' to do it. And with that you can be as brave or as stupid as you want to be. You have a choice of how far you push it, across both literal and metaphorical borders. Knowing when to step back and when to take up the responsibility and privilege we have been afforded to be able to tell these stories, to communicate the truth of the world around us. Do we go looking for the stories or do they find us, seek us out? It's my job to ask questions, sure, but I don't have all the answers. And I'm not for a moment comparing the experience of documenting the ruination of war to these stories, but there is something about the experience of being very close to another person's grief, that if you don't believe you are making a difference, it can be very destructive.

With that comes the questioning of ourselves, constantly: what is the best way to show you what I've seen? What I've heard? How do I ensure I'm telling you the 'truth'? Who is this for? You or for me? Does it help? Does it matter? I *hope* it does.

I ask Sam Peters this. He tells me if you're not telling people the truth, they cannot make an informed decision, and sport is filled with misinformation. Sam Peters has grasped the nettle hard, so to speak; he thinks this is, in part, because he knew he wouldn't be doing it for the rest of his life, that he could, in his own words, 'sacrifice myself on the altar of this' because he always had a plan at the back of his mind to move on to other things.

I think of him walking up the path to Laraine's house that day, about to drop a bombshell on the Astles, one that would not only change the course of their fight, but the fight of countless others. His sacrifice was worth it.

'He started telling us about all this that was going on in America with the NFL and all these former NFL players dying of this disease, CTE, chronic traumatic encephalopathy, which I'd never heard of. I could hardly say it, never mind understand what it meant!' Dawn laughs. 'And we were like, "Yeah?" Still thinking, "Why are you here?" And he said, "It's a 'brain disease." We were like, "Is it?" I['d] never heard of it.'

Peters told the Astles that CTE was not a new disease but that it used to be called boxer's brain, *dementia pugilistica* or punch drunk syndrome.

'And just for a split second, I was back in the coroner's court,' Dawn says, 'and I remembered Mr Robson describing my dad's brain as looking like the brain of a boxer. There was obviously something in my brain where it stored it,' she adds.

What followed was a conversation with Peters, who indicated that there are those who believe that perhaps footballers and rugby players are, through no fault of anybody, being misdiagnosed as having Alzheimer's, when in fact they could have this specific disease, which is caused by repeated blows to the head.

'So, I just asked him straight, I said, "My dad was diagnosed with Alzheimer's, do you think he might have had this disease, then?"' Dawn says. Sam Peters responded that it was a possibility. He gave Dawn the number of Dr Willie Stewart for her to follow up with.

'But then he started to ask about the FA and PFA research, and me and Mum were like, "Oh, yes, they're taking it very seriously." They started a study, and it's a longitudinal study. And this is 2014, so it was, like, 12 years ago, and we're thinking, *Oh, blimey, I wonder if it might be nearly finished now, this longitudinal study!*

'Sam Peters just sat there and said, "It hasn't been done."

'And I went, "You what?"' There's a quiet rage beneath Dawn's words.

'"I'm really sorry," Sam Peters said, "but I don't think it's been done."'

Dawn had a flurry of questions then. 'What do you mean it hasn't been done? Of course, it's been done! Are you sure?

Are you looking in the right places? Are you asking the right people?'

Sam Peters assured her, 'I wouldn't be here if I was getting any credible responses from anybody.' He had said, 'I'm hitting a wall of silence.'

Dawn was rocked by disbelief, which quickly transformed into anger.

'I kept saying, "Are you sure? Are you sure?"'

'Dawn, we can't find it,' Sam had said. 'Nobody will talk about it.'

For a moment Dawn could rationalise this in her head, concluding that there was no way the PFA would tell a reporter from the *Mail* about the study. Why would they trust him when it had nothing to do with him in the first place? He must have got it wrong. But then she looked over at Laraine who just said very quietly, 'I'm not surprised.'

Dawn tells me at that point you could have knocked her over with a feather. She was gobsmacked. Tears streamed down her face. She was angry, still in a state of disbelief, and she didn't know what to do then, who to call, who to email, how to get the answers for herself. She became hysterical, the grief of those 12 years coming upon her fast and hard. 'I was just saying, "Oh no, no, no, I need to—"' And then she left the house.[217]

Sam Peters describes Dawn as tenacious; he knew from their first encounter that here was someone who was going to cause the sports authorities quite a few problems, she wasn't going to go quietly. Having already been through the trauma of losing her father, the central figure in her life, in all their lives and as a much beloved player, they felt massively aggrieved. And they had every right to be.

'You know, some pretty powerful, important people have told them it was gonna be done and they've seen a coroner's report and all sorts of things that said, well, this is why he died, and this is what we think [about why] he died, so we'll look into it properly,' Sam Peters says.

It had given them a purpose for all those years, something to hold onto. Now here was the journalist telling them nothing had happened. Dawn left that conversation with Sam Peters and arrived home, still clutching the piece of paper with Dr Willie Stewart's number on it. She called him a few minutes after getting in and asked him to explain CTE.

She knew Laraine had donated Jeff's brain, but he had died 12 years prior to this conversation so she wasn't sure what could be done. Had the brain been kept? Would it disintegrate over time? Would it be too late to see if her father had the disease? Had he been misdiagnosed and if he had been, how many other footballers out there had been misdiagnosed too? Her mind was racing, but Dr Stewart was calm and reassuring.

'Yes, your father's brain should still be at Nottingham,' he had told her.[218]

'So, I spoke to Mum and she had no hesitation. I had no hesitation. My sisters had no hesitation to allow him to re-examine Dad's brain. It was no good to us. It was certainly no good to my dad. And if it would help other players and finally get some answers for us, it was absolutely, 100 per cent, the right thing to do,' Dawn says.

Sam Peters would run the story as part of a series of articles and investigations on concussion in the *Mail on Sunday* in 2014.[219] 'And you know, people accuse me of scaremongering and a lot worse,' he says. 'But I was convinced that it was the right path to go down.'[220]

They ran two stories initially; one was effectively a news story about how the PFA had failed to publish this research.[221] Peters and his colleagues reported that there was actually no evidence whatsoever that the study had ever been carried out. Gordon Taylor, the PFA chief executive at the time, insisted that 'there were some difficulties in keeping track of the individuals. But it was completed, although it hasn't been published.' And that it was still very much on the agenda and something he wanted to continue. 'We have had approaches from two hospitals with a view to continuing the studies.' Though no detail was given.

The article also details an encounter between Laraine Astle and former FA representative David Davies, a former BBC reporter who held executive positions at the FA from 1994 until 2007. Davies had visited her shortly after Jeff's death and promised to help her.

In his statement to the *Mail*, he is quoted as saying, 'I was always worried about this [the link between heading footballs and dementia]. I wish more could have been done. But it is entirely true that there was a view from some people that heading a ball, including those heavy footballs of days gone by, was part and parcel of the game.'[222]

***

Laraine Astle admits she isn't inclined to mess with technology, that frankly, she wouldn't even know how to plug a computer in, but tells me that Dawn and her younger sister started putting information out on Twitter and Facebook about the study not being done and that they wanted answers. This was soon picked up by a West Brom fan who printed out cards that gave all the details: in 2002 Jeff Astle had died and in 2014 the promised research hadn't been done. Why? Why did he die, aged 59? Why hadn't it mattered that the coroner said that football had killed him? Dawn and her sister handed them out at the West Brom home games with a group of volunteers. Dawn tells me that not a single one was dropped on the floor, screwed up or turned into a paper plane like most pamphlets in the stadium.

Their cause gathered momentum quickly with the backing of football fans; after all, fans never forget their old heroes. They had worshipped Jeff then and they worship him now. It culminated with a girl who had got in touch with an idea to put 'JUSTICE FOR JEFF' on big cards, and on the ninth minute of every match, because Jeff Astle was Number 9, they would hold them up in the stands.

It was seen on BBC's *Match of the Day* and Sky Live matches and the news spread even further.

They had a banner made, making the decision to take it to away matches.

'The first match we took it to was Hull away,' Dawn tells me. 'And Mum, bless her, because she's not online or anything, we gave her a specific job, and that was at the away games, she would ring the club and ask permission to bring this banner, and it was massive. It was sort of three-odd foot high and 30-odd foot long . . . it was . . . massive, [a] big heavy plasticky thing with "Justice For Jeff" on!'

Hull had no questions. They agreed instantly because they'd seen Sam Peters' stories in the *Mail on Sunday*.

'We took the banner, and on the ninth minute, we held it up, loads of us, because it was that long, and there was a minute's applause,' Dawn says, smiling.

They'd have it at the next home game, then the next away game, when they played Burnley, they asked again if they could take the banner. I smile at the thought of Laraine phoning the football clubs from her living room, the unofficial secretary of the campaign.

'And I'll never forget Burnley,' Dawn tells me. 'On the ninth minute, they put my dad's picture up on the electronic scoreboard and the whole place, wow, everybody was clapping. It was so moving. It's like people understood. This wasn't about making a name for ourselves. This wasn't about anything like that, about compensation, nothing. This was about getting the footballing authorities to do the right thing. Because people said to us, "Oh, what's the justice for?" And like, "The Justice for Jeff, what is it?"'[223]

'You look in the dictionary, there's lots of different meanings for justice, but this was about righting wrongs. It was wrong that they failed to do this research, they failed to do anything after this particular research collapsed after a few years. It was wrong that they never acknowledged what had happened to my dad and what had killed my dad. It was all about making sure that the right things were being done, not just to help former players in my dad's era, but for football's future.'[224]

The family seemed to amass an army behind them. Dawn recalls it feeling surreal. One minute they would all be sitting at home watching soaps and making dinner and the next minute, they were on *Good Morning Britain*, on national news and radio shows across the country. She admits it was terrifying to start with, having never done anything like that before in her life.

'Me and my sister [Claire] shook, like we literally shook every time and I always thought I was going to faint. You're so frightened of saying the wrong things and cocking it up with all these millions of listeners and people watching. We were just flung into the limelight, really.'[225]

It was in the papers virtually every week. It wasn't something that they had asked for, but it was something they felt they had to do.

And it is when I'm sitting on Dawn's sofa, cups of tea balancing, that she says to me, 'I promised my dad when I went to see him in the chapel of rest that if football was responsible and had killed him, I'd make sure the world knew about it, and I'd make sure something was done about it. I didn't want anybody else's dad to go through what we went through, and what my dad went through.'

Dawn and Claire would receive a lot of messages online – 'some real nasty ones' Laraine tells me, that would include things like, "He's in his box now, why are you bothering?"' Laraine was quite glad that she was sheltered from it by the girls, telling me that they would often come to a crisis point, questioning why they were putting themselves through this when there was nothing they could do to bring Jeff back.

But for every nasty message they received, there were so many brilliant ones, so many in fact that the family couldn't keep up. But these messages weren't just thank-yous or press requests. They were from former players' families saying: 'My dad's got dementia'; 'My dad died of dementia'; 'My husband died of dementia'; 'My husband's in a care home with dementia. He's only 63'; 'There's four from my dad's team. They're all in the same care home.' All of them were footballers.

'That was the turning point for me,' Dawn says. 'The families who came forward were so brave and so dignified ... without their coming forward, I would never, never have realised to what extent this dementia [existed] in football. I would never have realised.'

Dawn admits it was frightening, the idea that this could be just the tip of a massive iceberg, that there could be thousands of players suffering. She started to do her own research, gathering great longs lists with more names as more people got in touch. Occasionally it was one player out of the eleven on the team but then it wasn't, it was three out of the eleven, then five, then six. The list includes several members of the 1966 England World Cup team.

'And I thought, *Oh my God. This is massive,*' Dawn says. 'We've got to do something about this. This can't possibly be right. If football's killing all these players, I thought, they're going to have to do something. They're going to have to try and found out, have we got a problem? And that's the question I started to ask myself all the time: have we got a problem with our former players and dementia?'

Jeff Astle's case was not the first time neurodegenerative disease and the dangers of heading footballs had been presented to the Football Association (FA). In the 1990s, a decade before, Dr John Rowlands had begun to investigate football's problem with dementia. He had been alerted to the issue by the wife of a former player who was a family friend and a patient of his; her husband had passed away from Alzheimer's. It was an all too familiar story among the peers of her husband and she, quite rightly, wanted to investigate it, like Dawn. Dr Rowlands started to investigate, gathering material until he was convinced it was a problem. But if there's anything I've learnt, it doesn't matter how strong the evidence you amass, there are brick walls to be hit that will never come down.

In 1996, Dr Rowlands met with the PFA chief executive Gordon Taylor to inform him of what he perceived to be the problem. He was convinced it was the first time Taylor had heard of anything like it and remarked that he was extremely helpful in offering assistance to get the proposed research – a study in former players – off the ground, including support with funding.

Dr Rowlands sought the assistance of Dr Mark Doran, a neurology consultant, who prepared a detailed study which was titled, 'A proposal to determine the prevalence of dementia in professional footballers', but that's about as far as they would ever get.[226]

It's been widely that reported that Rowlands wrote to the FA following on from the conversation with Taylor and on 15 July 1996, he received a letter from Graham Kelly, then chief executive of the FA.[227] It thanks Rowlands for his letter, compliments his handwriting, which he notes is very good 'for a doctor', expresses his 'great interest' in the subject, with the promise of passing it on to the FA medical education department.

When Rowlands heard nothing further, he also wrote to Rick Parry, then chief executive of the Premier League. He received a response in October 1996 from secretary Mike Foster, who wrote: 'Mr Parry has passed on to me a copy of your letter. I have to inform you that the Premier League does not have any specific funds available for this purpose.'[228]

Rowlands continued to write to the major clubs in England, but to no avail. He's not the only one. Dr Mike Sadler was interviewed by various news outlets stating that he too tried to raise the issue in letters to PFA chief executive Gordon Taylor between 1993 and 1997.

As a very keen football fan, and a doctor, he had noted the number of former players who seemed to develop neurological disease prematurely, with examples such as Danny Blanchflower,

Ray Kennedy and Bob Paisley, the latter of whom he had met when his illness had started to become evident.

'It seemed to me that this could relate to multiple head trauma, from both heading and direct contact during the game, and [so I] discussed this with Kevin Moore, the Saints captain who I knew well at that time,' Sadler said. Moore agreed that someone in his position suffered multiple trauma to the head during a game, and that this issue would be worth exploring.

'I initially wrote to Gordon Taylor directly, in late 1993, early 1994, suggesting a study comparing former players, with goal-keepers as a comparative subset of footballers who didn't routinely head the ball, with the general population. I received a fairly dismissive reply from Gordon Taylor, saying that the PFA didn't keep records that would enable this study, but offering no other thoughts or encouragement.'

Through a friend, Mike Sadler was able to ask Iain Dowie, then a Saints PFA rep, to take a letter to the next PFA meeting, which he did, but again without positive response.

Sadler said, 'Without the co-operation of the PFA, it was hard to pursue this theory at that time, but then in 1997, the Lancet published a paper showing brain injury in footballers, thought to be due to repeated head trauma, so I wrote to Gordon Taylor again, but without response.'[229]

Sadler tells me that although he's happy that the work has continued, and although we are slightly more informed, he is also frustrated.

'In 1994, if we had done a ten-year study, that would have ended 17 years ago and we would have much more data about the people that are particularly at risk and why that is and done the appropriate further studies based on what was found.'

Instead, Sadler thinks that we haven't really moved on and considers the 28 years a wasted opportunity for progress and ultimately safety.

It has been widely reported that Taylor denied ignoring the issue and has said that he does not know of any other football organisation in the world that has done more than the PFA.

'We are aware of the literally dozens of research projects throughout the world on this issue,' he has said. 'No causal link has yet been established between heading the ball and various neurological problems such as dementia and CTE.'[230]

But a link had been considered long before then, in 1984, when a medical article written by Vojin N. Smodlaka, a professor for rehabilitation medicine at the State University of New York College of Medicine in Brooklyn, was published in the magazine of World Governing Body FIFA, highlighting the dangers of heading the ball.

The article is titled 'How dangerous is heading?' and across the two pages of text, it discusses the possibility of CTE, stating, 'Heading the ball causes a significant blow to the head,' and 'the only protection is to decrease the number of headings.'

The article concludes:

The sports medicine community has not devoted enough attention to this important problem of possible brain damage. When an athlete is knocked down and is unconscious for several seconds during a competition, in many cases he or she will be allowed to immediately continue the game but, if an athlete sustains a sprain or strain, they will stop. The sports community must take brain concussions more seriously.[231]

In 2000, the year prior to the study and two years prior to Jeff Astle's death, the BBC reported 'Head Injury Plea to Footballers', which detailed a warning from the Scottish Professional Footballers Association calling on footballers to register their head injuries following concern that they could lead to problems later in life. The concern came as a result of Celtic player Bill McPhail being diagnosed with pre-senile dementia, which he blamed on heading footballs, and subsequently launching a legal case in 1999 claiming that he was entitled to disability payments, though an industrial tribunal did not accept that a clash of heads during his playing career could have caused the dementia.[232]

In an interview with BBC *Frontline Scotland*'s 'Heading for Trouble' programme broadcast on 2 May 2000, his wife Ophelia had said: 'Somebody should be responsible for an accident that happens at work, and I think football has always turned its back on these players.'[233]

They were not successful.

'The industrial tribunal didn't accept that the head knocks during his playing career could have caused the dementia which Billy began showing signs of in his thirties,' Ophelia tells the reporter Jane Frachi in the programme. 'His lawyer knows that establishing that link is going to be an uphill struggle.'

At that point heading the ball was categorised as part of the job [as a footballer] and not an industrial injury. The decision was upheld by the Social Security Commissioner of Scotland.[234]

The programme also featured another former Celtic player, Jock Weir, who had been suffering from a similar illness. The descriptions from both players' wives are eerily similar to how Dawn and Laraine Astle have detailed Jeff's experience in our conversations.

The programme concludes that though there was a lot of evidence to support the relationship between heading and dementia, the jury was still out on a definitive link.[235] It is interesting to me that the dialogue had started prior to Jeff Astle and on a public platform like the BBC. But it seems that serious attention was not paid until the Astle's Justice for Jeff campaign started.

The campaign culminated in the Astle family being told that while the FA and PFA had jointly commissioned a study in 2001, which tracked 32 professional footballers under the age of 20 over a ten-year period, it was ultimately deemed inconclusive. It had ended after five years, though this wasn't made clear to the public.

Greg Dyke was the FA chairman at the time, and publicly vowed there would be no repeat of the FA's failure to deliver potentially life-saving research into links between concussion and early-onset dementia. He admitted that his organisation's response to Jeff Astle's death was 'woefully inadequate'.[236]

'We promised the Astle family we would do some research and we didn't, and that is a failure by the FA and, yes, we are now going to do it,' he told the *Mail on Sunday*.[237]

This was the first open admission that the study wasn't completed. I put it to the FA, asking for more detail, and while the request was acknowledged by a representative, no further detail has since been provided. Though they are making moves now, which I'll come back to later.

But at this time the Astle family wanted answers. They wanted to know why the study hadn't been finished and more importantly why they weren't told until years later.

'And I've always said ... we've always known, at the beginning, they shied away from it, because it was, "Oh. The national game." Nobody wanted to see anything bad in it,' Laraine Astle says. 'But we knew that we had a cause. We knew the truth.'[238]

They also knew that Jeff's brain had been re-examined.

'It was relatively easy for us because we knew that's what Dad believed in, he didn't have opinions on much apart from football, cricket and horseracing, but he did really believe in organ donation,' Dawn tells me. 'And it's a good job we did it because I wouldn't be talking to you now! I wouldn't be! Hang on, let me find the letter ...' she says, rummaging in a cupboard.

'Got it! It's a bit lengthy but this is a segment that I ...' she stops abruptly. 'God, I think this is going to upset me, reading this now.' I can hear the crack in her voice.

It's a letter from the Queen's Medical Centre in Nottingham where they had donated Jeff's brain for research. The letter is sincere, expressing thanks to the whole family for the donation, for providing another piece in a jigsaw to help build and complete the picture of how the brain works and for their willingness to try to make a better future for other people. It was a valuable gift for future generations.

Dawn reads it to me but stops abruptly on finishing. 'Oh God! Bloody hell!' She is audibly upset now. She exhales and I wait. 'Little did we know when we did donate Dad's brain that it would help! That it would reveal what it did.'

Little did she know that it would be the catalyst for everything.

In 2014, Dawn picked up Dr Willie Stewart from East Midlands Airport. He had flown in from Scotland to give the diagnosis of Jeff's brain in person and the two of them drove to Laraine's, where he told them he had indeed found CTE.

'Now, I'd like to think I'm reasonably intelligent, but I didn't understand a word he was on about!' Dawn says, laughing. 'He was talking about this, that and the other, and the odd word I recognised, but I didn't understand him. He's a scientist and an incredibly intelligent man who's devoted his life to looking at the brain, and I didn't know what he was on about!'

She asked Dr Stewart to explain to them in layman's terms what the disease is and what was happening. He told them that CTE is a form of dementia that's progressive, that there's no cure and the signs and symptoms are very, very similar to Alzheimer's. But they're caused by repeated blows to the head, repeated concussions or repeated subconcussive blows. That could translate to an elbow to the head, while Jeff was playing, kicks to the head or, like the coroner had said, the repeated heading of a football over a 15-odd-year career.

'And he started to talk about the ball and what happens to the brain, and I was getting all confused again, and I said, "Woah, woah, woah, just explain to me very simply, please!"'

Dr Stewart asked her to imagine that a ball was being kicked at her. 'Would you use your laptop or your plasma TV screen or your LCD screen as a bat?' he'd said.

'I said, "Well, no. Course I wouldn't."'

'Well, why wouldn't you?' he asked.

'Well, you'd smash the screen,' Dawn said.

'Exactly. So, when you look down at that smashed screen, you'll see on the floor hundreds, perhaps thousands of tiny fragments of glass or plastic. So, what is that doing to the most fragile, the most complex, the most unique organ in the body, the brain?'

Dawn was stunned. More so when he told her that her father's was the worst case of CTE he had ever seen and if he hadn't known he was looking at the brain of a 59-year-old man, he'd have thought he was looking at a brain of a man well into his nineties. It was difficult for the family to grasp. Why had Jeff Astle died of boxer's brain when he was a footballer?

The re-examination of the brain took things to another level because in the same way that Mike Webster became the first NFL player to be diagnosed with CTE, Jeff Astle became the first British footballer to be confirmed as dying of CTE. It was fortunate that Laraine had had the foresight to donate Jeff's brain, otherwise there would never have been the evidence. You can't argue with the evidence; the brain showed why Jeff had what he had. Why he'd died of what he died of. It was there for all to see. Here was the proof.

The results of Jeff Astle's brain diagnosis in 2014 came the same year that the NFL agreed to pay a class-action lawsuit that had been filed on behalf of more than 4,500 ex-players in 2012. The settlement was US $765 million.[239] The final agreement allowed for up to US $1 billion in compensation for retired players with serious medical conditions linked to repeated head trauma. Both felt like enormous turning points but there was an eery period of calm that followed them: the subject of concussion and CTE seemed to disappear from UK football as it had seemingly disappeared from the NFL narrative. Perhaps it was an assumption that since the NFL's $765 million settlement had passed, the game was now safer.

In reality, the NFL never truly accepted liability for anything, and have long denied any wrongdoing, and insisted that safety always has been a top priority.[240]

'This agreement lets us help those who need it most and continue our work to make the game safer for current and future players. Commissioner Goodell and every owner gave the legal team the same direction: do the right thing for the game and for the men who played it,' said NFL Executive Vice President Jeffrey Pash. 'We thought it was critical to get more help to players and families who deserve it, rather than spend many years and millions of dollars on litigation. This is an important step that builds on the significant changes we've made in recent years to make the game safer, and we will continue our work to better the long-term health and wellbeing of NFL players.'[241]

In the days following, Goodell reiterated that, 'There was no admission that anything was caused by football.'[242]

According to data compiled and analysed by IQVIA, an independent third-party company retained by the NFL, the sport has succeeded in reducing concussions, which were at their highest number in 2017 at a total of 281 for pre-season and regular season. Despite changing the rules to allow for more severe penalties and fines for deliberate helmet-to-helmet hits, the number of concussions sustained during practice and gameplay increased in 2019 to 224 from a previous 214 in 2018. But in 2020 the number of reported concussions decreased once again to 172.[243]

This data doesn't cover the additional blows to the head that don't reach the level of concussion but still may pose a risk for the brain. Injury rates between games has increased since 2017.

To the average American football fan and average American football player, it seems that the game is safer, and while elements of it are, the players are still at risk. They've been lulled into a false sense of security that there is nothing to be worried about now.

There are heroes and villains in every story worth telling, although in this case it's not so black and white, especially when everyone believes that they are on the side of progress. Many researchers are united in their belief that it is a moral compass that skews the focus. Very simply, you're either doing what is right in this discussion or you're not. It feels like the multi-million-dollar lawsuit actually worked in the NFL's favour, that the amount of money overshadowed the actual reality of what was happening and the reason it was being paid out – that players were suffering or dying. It seems to have been a mastermind of a PR campaign to cover up injuries you can't see. But they are still there – only just under the surface.

'You know at some point somebody figured out that the long-term risk issue was a threat to the finances of their sport,' Chris Nowinski says. 'And, you know, it still shocks me that CTE was discovered in boxers and no one questions it. And they literally have ice hockey players playing like boxers on skates pretending like that's a different risk! That's insane to me!'[244]

I wonder how sport gets away with it but then I think back to the cricket match in Korail, to the hundreds of people not only captivated by sport but united in their community, in the possibility of a future because of it. That hope is intoxicating.

'People are conforming to a cast of the mind which has been fed to them by propaganda like Fox News. So they belong to a group, a way of thinking; an intelligence of the individual is being controlled by the expectation of the larger group and you become embedded, you become absorbed, almost becoming irrational,' says Dr Bennet Omalu.

There are those that think the football industry has done a brilliant job in permeating the entire fabric of American society so that Americans believe that football is what defines their country. The Super Bowl Sunday is almost as big a holiday as Independence Day, which ultimately means the NFL now owns a day of the year.

On the flip side are the NFL, FA, PFA, AFL, and other such sports organisations, serving at the pleasure of the people; they need the public's support – and it's been public pressure and campaigning that have led to a real change in the way dementia, concussion, CTE and sports have been viewed.

In 2017, following 18 months of relentless campaigning by the English newspaper the *Telegraph*, the PFA agreed to commission a study into the link between football and dementia after the paper sought to expose what had been branded sport's 'silent scandal'.[245] The study intended to compare the causes of death of 7,676 former Scottish male professional football players who were born between 1900 and 1976 against those of more than 23,000 matched individuals from the general population. The study would be led by Dr Willie Stewart who would essentially build on the study format that Dr Rowlands had, unbeknownst to him, proposed all those years before.

The results came out in autumn 2019 and found, in short, that professional footballers had approximately three and a half times higher rates of death due to neurodegenerative diseases than the general population.[246]

It's important to note that although footballers have this higher risk factor, they are less likely to die of other common diseases, such as heart disease and some cancers, including lung cancer.

Dr Stewart stated, 'While every effort must be made to identify the factors contributing to the increased risk of neurodegenerative disease to allow this risk to be reduced, there are also wider potential health benefits of playing football to be considered.'[247]

The PFA released a statement that detailed their commitment to doing everything they could to support any members dealing with dementia, and their families. They extended their support with a detailed plan that had points of action, including:

- a dementia helpline in partnership with the Alzheimer's Society, available for PFA members,
- continued support for members who received a diagnosis of dementia,
- a call-out to FIFA, FIFAPro, UEFA, the Premier League and EFL, to join them in determining how the industry will protect its current players and support former players.
- a football-wide fund for dementia,
- precautionary changes that may help minimise potential risks, including:
    - adapting training schedules to reduce the frequency of heading the ball.
    - strengthen concussion protocol and management of head injuries.
    - introduce new rules, such as the use of concussion sub-stitutions.

They also committed to further research so they could effectively advocate on their members' behalf to the governing bodies of the sport and make informed decisions about effectively reducing risk factors. They also stated that as part of the longitudinal aspect of these studies, brain donations from former professional footballers would be required after death for autopsy.

I emailed Dawn immediately on seeing the results sweep across social media like a tidal wave. For such a long time the Astle family were the lone voices on this, but Dawn knew that one day she would be proved right, though the results were bittersweet.

'I mean, there was no celebration, nobody was punching the air thinking, *Yes we were right, we showed them we were right, we were right all along!* There was none of that,' Dawn says. 'It was just sadness really because the figures are shocking. But I wasn't particularly shocked because I knew it, I knew. I would have been more shocked if it wasn't.'

Dawn has been around the block enough times to know that just because something was said, even in the public domain, it didn't mean things would get done.

'This just feels like the end of the first chapter,' she said. 'We're about to start chapter two.'

Why is she so tentative? Because while it can be seen as a victory for the families concerned, the question remains: why has it taken over 25 years for this to happen when the warning signs, material and awareness from medics and the PFA alike have been there all along? It's what happens next that really matters.

'CTE is an inconvenient truth for everyone,' Dr Omalu told me when we spoke in 2018, 'but the truth is the truth.' A truth that Dr Omalu is convinced will ultimately prevail, that humanity will surpass any corporate interest, that human beings come first and, in his own words, that 'the humanity of football surpasses the business of football'.

You have to admire his optimism. I wasn't sure, but then again at least brain injury gained a presence within sport. It was at least being discussed and researched and debated. Yet there are more vulnerable groups where the discourse around CTE and certainly traumatic brain injury is practically non-existent.

One of those groups is women.

'Is this football town putting its daughters at risk to protect its sons?'[248]

— Rachel Dissell, *Cleveland Plain Dealer* journalist

Trigger Warning: This chapter contains detailed discussion of domestic abuse and violence against women.

Chapter Eight
The War Zone

Ella's eyes dart to the door every time an unexpected sound interrupts our conversation.

An instep she doesn't recognise on the pavement, a car door shut with unfamiliar force, a child's gleeful 'GO FAAAASTER!' rebounding off the window as they whizz past the house on their bike.

'Force of habit!' She catches me and rolls her eyes into a smile.

Both her hands were balled into fists when I came in, but they're now unfurled. I notice half-moons hollowed across her palms where her nails have been holding in her nerves. She lets my questions steep, chewing over the words like toffee before she decides on her answer, swallowing the hard parts back down until she trusts me completely. She's cautious, of course, but she isn't scared.

'Have you ever been in love?' she asks, clasping her hands back together. 'Have you ever been so fucking crazy in love that you've sort of. . .' She trails off, eyes rolling again, hands suddenly reaching towards her temples as she mimes what I can loosely interpret as 'lost your mind'.

'I have,' I say.

A breath. A beat.

'And what's weird is that I always thought this was so protected,' she says, tapping her skull gently with her finger. 'I wonder if he had known the damage it would cause, if I had known. Whether it might have made a difference.'

She looks at me momentarily for reassurance before deciding for herself. 'You don't think how much your head, you know, brain, can be affected by an impact which you know happens so quickly and then obviously your bruises heal, and you seem to feel OK. Looking back, it does make a lot of sense as to why I don't have any short-term memory and it's due to the actions of someone, you know, doing what they did.'[249]

★★★

In the build-up to the 2017 Super Bowl, the *US Vogue* Instagram account posted an image by Irving Penn, titled 'Football Face, New York'.[250] They posted it again in 2020 and 2021.[251] If you're unfamiliar with the image, it's a photograph of a woman with her bare shoulders hunched forward – a posture that indicates both her age (young, naive) and accentuates her frame (slender, bony, ideal).

Her head is cocked to one side, wisps of loose blonde curls frame her face. It's that sexy, doesn't-try-hard hairstyle that magazines tell women men love.

189

Only, this woman doesn't have a face. Instead, her features have been replaced by the stitches and deflated skin of an American football; dark brown leather pieces haphazardly sewn together with thick white thread that starts where her nose should be and tracks all the way up to her hairline.

Her mouth, unsurprisingly, has been completely covered.

It's a disturbing image, risqué, grotesque even. It stopped my scroll in its tracks and I wasn't the only one. An onslaught of comments quickly appeared, ranging from, 'I don't know how to feel about this', to 'creepiest image I've ever seen' and then later, 'I can't believe this is still up. Unfollow.'

I couldn't believe it myself.

Not because of the violence of the image, but that it was being used by *Vogue* to mark the Super Bowl.

There are also comments that argue it's 'art', alongside cries of, 'Don't listen to them! It's stunning.' The image was divisive, that was clear: a beauty and a beast.

Penn himself had once said that he recognised the camera 'for the instrument it is, part Stradivarius, part scalpel'.[252] There was one comment under the post that stood out to me the most: 'Who's the poor victim in this photo?'[253]

It's one of the details that I can recall vividly. There are others – sights and scents and scenes that roll to the front of my mind, not particularly in order but I have come to learn that this is how memory works. Our brain stores a series of brief fleeting moments – visual snapshots, sounds, smells, thoughts and feelings – and each time we remember, we piece these together to create an episodic memory of an event. These events in turn can be used to build up a narrative of a whole day or even a whole lifetime.

Memories are not constructed from precise records of what actually happened – but rather from records of what we experienced. Imagine them as piles of Polaroids strewn out on a coffee table. Some are buried underneath the pile, some have been scattered onto the floor below, perhaps floated under a sofa, or down the cracks of a floorboard, forgotten for a time. Memories associated with grief or trauma will usually find their way to the surface.

The image by Penn is one of those, or more poignantly, the fact that it felt so fateful to my work is one of those. That he had chosen a football to cover the woman's face. It was a perfect metaphor for explaining what is happening with research into traumatic brain injury (TBI); that women have not only been overshadowed by sport, but left out of the conversation almost entirely.

That's not a new phenomenon, women have historically been left out of medical research.

It was only in 1994 that the National Institutes of Health mandated the inclusion of women in clinical trials. For context, that was also the year *Friends* first debuted on television, the year Tom Hanks won his second Oscar for *Forrest Gump*, and the year I'd put on a school uniform for the first time.

There were three resounding reasons for this exclusion: the first was due to concerns about a woman's exposure to risk during childbearing years; the second, because of misperceptions that treatment was the same across sex and gender; and the third was a belief that women's menstrual and hormone cycles would bring unnecessary complications.

In essence, the fault was our own for being women.

Worldwide, women with dementia outnumber men two to one. Dementia and the prevalence and life-time risk of Alzheimer's disease is higher in females than in males and yet the field of brain injury in sport continues to be dominated by sports concussion research on male athletes and traditionally male sports.

Most of what people know about traumatic brain injuries and their side effects comes from studies of male veterans, football players, ice hockey players, despite an increasing number of women stepping into those arenas who play with the same ferocity as their male counterparts. Research suggests that not only are female athletes more likely to sustain a concussion in any given sport; they also tend to have more severe symptoms and take longer to recover.[254] A study of 266 adolescents – including European football and American football players, wrestlers and skiers – found that, on average, women took 76 days to recover, while men took 50.[255] There are reasons as to why this might be though none of them are fully backed up due to a lack of research.

Some researchers have stated that anatomical differences in the male and female body and brain are contributing factors, along with varying female hormone levels during the menstrual cycle, which can affect the risk and recovery of concussion.

Researchers at the University of Rochester School of Medicine and Dentistry tracked the progress of 144 concussed women, visiting six emergency departments in upstate New York and Pennsylvania, and found that injuries sustained after menstruation and before ovulation were less likely to lead to symptoms a month later, while an injury that occurred after ovulation and before menstruation resulted in significantly worse outcomes.[256]

It's still unclear as to why that is. Then there are some that suggest many of the reported sex differences are simply the result of societal gender roles. While men have been conditioned to play through pain, women have been considered more honest about their injuries.

I spoke to coaches and researchers, who offered some explanation as to why this is. As women's sports have gained recognition, being elevated to primetime spots on television networks like Women's Football on the BBC, the pressure to perform as trailblazers, to pave the way for other women to come through, coupled with the added weight of the women that went before that didn't get the same platform, means that they remain tight-lipped and won't go on the record for research projects. The coaches had it on good authority that women didn't want to be seen as troublemakers, that they had fought so long to be considered equal to their male counterparts yet still felt powerless, as if everything they had built could crumble at any second and their careers be taken away. There are some who have spoken openly, but often they are sportswomen who have made the big time. The American World Cup-winning team players, for example, have been vocal about their concussions.

Even the brain banks across the globe house tissue from an overriding majority of male brains. At the time of writing this, in 2021, the Boston University Brain Bank houses over 800 brains including over 320 with CTE. Of those only a tiny percentage (about 6 per cent) are from women.

The common term associated with women and concussion is TBI – traumatic brain injury – which is defined as 'an alteration in brain function or other evidence of brain pathology caused by an external force'.[257] An external force like a boxing glove, a football or a fist.

This brings me back to Penn's image. There was something about the horror of it, the violence of the stitches, the worn leather stretched across her mouth that makes her faceless, silent. She can be anyone or anything. And what is it that men do on a football field with balls like that? They kick them, throw them, bat them. She looks like a punching bag.

It is this interpretation of Penn's image that overrides the rest for me, the one that remains at the forefront of my mind. There are others too, the ones that I can reach for without effort that have become imprinted somehow, like the unusual pattern of the chunky knit jumper Dr John Hardy was wearing the day he handed me the research papers on 'The Punch Drunk Wife'.[258] Dr Hardy is chair of Molecular Biology of Neurological Disease at University College London's Institute of Neurology.

In the doctor's case, not only did the loudness of his patterned knitwear silence the sea of science researchers we had walked through at UCL, but it filled the glass room we found ourselves in with a warmth and sense of humour that meant flicking through the images of a woman's battered brain became a fraction more bearable. A fraction.

I have often thought perhaps it was a conscious decision on the part of Hardy, a talking point to distract the eyes and mind from the disturbance that was to follow; scanned images of a real human brain full of tears and holes to illustrate the paper's vivid descriptions of abuse that subsequently ended up in a devastating diagnosis. Once you have seen something like that, you cannot unsee it, brain scan and knitwear alike. We laughed about the jumper in the same breath that we established CTE was absolutely an outcome of domestic violence.

'This is boxing! This is boxing,' Dr Hardy had repeated, as if he could not quite believe it himself. I had had the inclination early on: that if heading a football, taking a hit from a boxing glove or clashing heads on an NFL field caused this disease, then what about the over one in three women who are

experiencing intimate partner violence, who are being repeatedly struck on the head?

This hunch had led me to Dr John Hardy at UCL, who
handed over a 1990 scientific study conducted by Dr Gareth
Roberts, titled 'Dementia in a Punch-Drunk Wife'.[259] This was
one of the first cases of CTE to ever be reported in a woman.
The so-called 'Punch-Drunk Wife' was a 76-year-old woman
who endured a history of violent abuse at the hands of her husband and had become 'demented over her last few years'. After
her death, the report revealed 'abnormal thickening of the ears,
resembling the cauliflower ears of pugilists'.

Boxers.

On the face of it boxing and domestic violence are likely
medical pairings, particularly given what we now know
about repetitive impacts to the head. Despite the similarities
in exposure, the two have never been treated in the same
way. Safety in boxing would ultimately end up in the House
of Lords, where the invisible epidemic of violence against
women was silenced by shame. The only real difference is
gender.

In their recent study, Stephen Caspar and Kelly O'Donnell
state that in the matter of traumatic head injury, women are
expected to experience assault as an acute episode, followed by
chronic emotional disturbance. Boxers, usually men, were denied
chronic emotional disturbance and permitted brain injury as a
consequence. It's taken years to grasp that the visible problems
of athletes are really invisible injuries, the consequences of their
repeated assaults, so what chance does a battered woman have?

The term 'battered' first appeared in a pioneering study in
1968, which combined social work and psychiatric theory
to examine the psychical dimensions of child abuse.[260] It was

co-opted as clinical language in 1975 by J.J. Gayford as a way to describe case studies of violence in the home and 'battered women's syndrome'. There is one line that really stands out to me, when a victim states that most of the bruises had been done to her scalp 'where they do not show'. There has been research that shows that a lot of abusers are getting smarter about how to engage in violent encounters without leaving marks, without bruising, hit behind the hairline, for example, and strangulation up to a point that doesn't leave visible marks. It means that women are being seen by police officers or entering emergency rooms where treating physicians can't see any visible damage. Ninety per cent of violent encounters include hits to the head, face and neck, including strangulation, all of which are likely to be able to cause a traumatic brain injury either through direct impact or shaking. Even if somebody is thrown, that can easily result in damage to the axonal shearing, which is a stretching of sort of the pathways in the brain that transmit information.

Part of the challenge with concussive injury and mild-to-moderate traumatic brain injury is that it's cumulative. One injury is one injury and then the next one might be two, but, when you're starting to talk about maybe five injuries or six, adding up on top of each other, the amount of challenge and resulting difficulties for each injury can get bigger and bigger, and more problematic, and more difficult to pinpoint, so you can end up with really significant post-injury difficulties from what people might think of as a relatively minor incident.

Overall, 70 per cent of the TBI population is made up of men. There are a variety of reasons for that, which have to do with things like general activities and perhaps testosterone and reckless behaviour in youth, that kind of thing. So, there's been more men to do research on than there have been women.

Historically, medical research in general has focused on males, right down to basic science where the lab rats tend to be male rats.

It's only recently that medicine has started to recognise that this is a flawed approach and results in male-dominated data and in a male-dominated understanding of the condition. It is moving towards a gender difference in healthcare research and the experiences of survivors.

When I was a child, I had a box of puppets and an enormous, fold-out cardboard booth which I stored under my bed. It was painted with bright stripes, reminiscent of the classic *Punch and Judy* booths we had seen at village fêtes or by the seaside. My puppets weren't as terrifying as the classic 'Punch', with his bulbous whisky-blushed nose and pointed chin. Occasionally, a Teenage Mutant Ninja Turtle would take his place and save the day, or if my younger brother, bored and irritated with my script that he couldn't yet read, decided to go off-piste, we could end up with a 'Hot Wheels Micro-Car' speed chase or an unrehearsed made-up song with 'poo' in the title or the whole place would start raining Duplo blocks, ultimately leaving the cardboard flattened and me wailing in despair.

Occasionally we'd get our acts together, mimicking the *Punch and Judy* shows we'd seen at our village schools. Punch was always the hero. We'd meet him first as he is waiting for Judy, who had been cooking the dinner or tending to their baby, busying herself with the stuff that wives do. He was likely drunk, bowling around the booth, his face red and blotchy eyes wild, nose and chin like the Child Catcher from *Chitty Chitty Bang Bang*. He would be calling for Judy who would often appear after he'd had his first few minutes of fame, clutching either a string of sausages or the baby or both, to our wild amusement. They would begin their slapstick back and forth, a knock here, a slap there, sometimes there were sound effects, a kazoo for comedic effect, the perfectly timed ba-dum-tss of a drum kit as one of them was knocked out with a stick. The poor baby didn't last long either, making a swift exit stage left or being hurled from the booth after an altercation with either parent. On occasion, the baby would be turned into a sausage, much to our delight. A policeman might arrive to see what all the fuss was about, we'd shout at him under the instruction of Punch. Nothing to see here officer. The bumbling police officer would fall foul of the slapstick too; a crocodile might arrive and nip everyone where it shouldn't, and we would laugh and laugh. With everyone out of the way and suitably entertained, Punch would then turn his attention to Judy and club her to death, squeaking 'that's the way to do it' before bowing to roaring applause.

It was all fun and games.

Investigating something like this changes the way you see things. I was rewatching an episode of *Friends*, when the untrained, unexpectant Ross Geller, a lanky, goofy but ultimately lovable palaeontologist, finds himself in a game of rugby with the English friends of the woman he is dating. Men that are much bigger, stockier and stereotypically more masculine than the PhD palaeontologist. They destroy him in a game that leaves him broken and bloody. The canned laughter roars throughout his demise, which veers towards slapstick. And though I'm not suggesting that it was a deliberate decision on the part of the writers or producers to present the injury in this way, it feels uncomfortable to me now. I see it differently.

In reference to symptoms, in season eight of another comedy show, *Modern Family*, a player on the college football team is left with a head injury following a game and remarks to the team, 'Can anybody else see that giant chicken or is it just me?' as he stands swaying, dazed and confused. Once again, the canned laugher is right on cue. It's nothing new, we've seen it in cartoons for decades and decades – the swirling ring of stars above Tom and Jerry's heads after their opponent has taken a mallet to their skull. They're stopped in their tracks for a second until the spinning subsides and then it's back to play. Violence in cartoons is an integral part of its content. Researchers Potter and Warren found, in 1998, that the frequency of violence in cartoons is higher than in live-action dramas or comedies.[261] Which means that young people are more likely to view media-depicted violence during a Saturday-morning cartoon than during primetime adult television hours in the evening. There are differences between those acts of violence: cartoon violence is meant for a young audience and is more likely to involve minor acts that are not realistic. Death is rarely shown with cartoons, which sanitise the outcomes of violence, showing a full recovery after a huge blow to the head. It is very unusual to see the victims suffering in a lifelike manner.

The presence or absence of comedy during violence was found to be an important consideration when evaluating the effects of viewing cartoons on young people, for there is both theory and research to support the contention that comedic elements may camouflage and trivialise depictions of violence.[262] For instance, in a research project for *Journalism Quarterly* in 1974, R.P. Snow had young people evaluate cartoons, live-action dramas and news footage of the Vietnam War for presence of violence.[263] The young people would consistently overlook the violent elements in the cartoons with only 27 per cent of the children aged between four and eight, and 16 per cen of those aged between nine and twelve, correctly identifying that the cartoon (i.e. *Roadrunner*) contained violence. In comparison, nearly 70 per cent of the young people in Snow's sample classified the television Western *Gunsmoke* as containing violence. Regardless of age, all children correctly identified news clips of the Vietnam War as containing violent imagery.[264]

I'm not going to make a tenuous link between the violence in the cartoons and the behaviour of children. I'm not a psychologist. But like with anything as we are growing up, we absorb, we desensitise, and we copy what we see. Whether that's donning a cape and running around the backyard as Batman or pulling a football shirt over the top of our heads when we score a goal. Our lives are shaped by the world around us and if there is no one to educate us, to warn us, what happens then?

We wouldn't sit a child in front of images of the Vietnam War on a Saturday morning, but if violence slips through the net under the guise of comedy, exhibited by our favourite brightly coloured animations, then we imprint on young people early on that it's just a bump or a knock. I have to question whether the reluctance for anyone to acknowledge the severity of head injury hasn't been engraved from factors other than just sport, so I can't discount these early interactions.

***

In the mid-1990s, Dr Eve Valera was a graduate student, volunteering at a domestic violence shelter. She was also actively obtaining training in neuropsychology and came to wonder about the rates and effects of traumatic brain injuries in women experiencing violence in this way. She was stunned when, after a thorough literature search, she failed to find any articles addressing the topic. She knew there had to be a connection.

I met Dr Valera while researching the documentary *The Beautiful Brain* in 2019, after my own hunch about domestic violence led me down the same route. Through a daisy chain of contributors, I was finally sent her way.

In 2003, alongside Howard Berenbaum, Dr Valera had conducted a study titled 'Brain Injury in Battered Women'.[265] The goals of the study were to examine:

(a) whether battered women in a sample of both shelter and non-shelter groups were sustaining brain injuries from their partners; and

(b) if so, whether such brain injuries were associated with partner abuse severity, cognitive functioning or psychopathology.

Eve Valera is sharp as a dart and talks quickly and assertively: 'So, the first work that I did was actually using neuropsychological measures, interview measures and basically asking women questions that would get at whether or not they sustained brain injuries, even if they didn't necessarily recognise that that's what was going on. Because a lot of people don't necessarily recognise that.

'Now, people may be a little more aware because of all the media attention with athletics and the military chronic traumatic encephalopathy. So, all of that stuff has raised a little bit more awareness about concussion and what can cause a concussion and what a concussion may mean, although there's still a ton of confusion over what that means.'

Typically, women don't think anything of it, especially if they have other things to deal with, like a broken hand or if their ear is bleeding.

'Or their eye socket is hanging off,' Valera offers. 'It sounds gross, but these are things that actually happen,' she says.

If things like that occur, people often go to hospital.

'But with respect to a hit on the head or if they're smashed against the wall, have their head stomped, whatever, and then they either lose consciousness or don't remember part of it or are really dazed or confused and disoriented, the women that I spoke to really don't go to the hospital for that. I can't remember one woman who said, "Yeah, that happened to me, so I went to the hospital to get it checked out." If they do go, it's for other stuff,' she says.[256]

Later, in 2017, Valera revisited this research and with Aaron Kucyi conducted a new study which formed the basis of 'Brain injury in women experiencing intimate partner-violence: neural mechanistic evidence of an invisible trauma'.[267]

The participants of this study were 20 women recruited from women's shelters, domestic violence programmes and by word-of-mouth. Similar to the first study, a history of non-partner and partner-related TBI was assessed in the group.[268]

During the study, Valera asked the women the following questions: 'After anything your partner ever did to you, did you ever lose consciousness or black out?' 'After anything your partner did to you, did you not remember a certain part around that incident?' or 'Did you ever feel really dazed, confused, or disoriented?' And if they responded 'yes', then she would say, 'OK, can you tell me what happened?'

And ask if what had happened was the result of their head being stomped on or smashed against the wall or a floor? Or if they been thrown downstairs or steps? And then if, for a period of time they experienced the aforementioned symptoms, then that was identified as a concussion or a mild traumatic brain injury.

'That's basically what I did to get the information . . . then I related, well, I got the incidents of that, then I related that to measures of cognitive functioning by using neuropsychological tests that measure things like memory, working, cognitive flexibility. And then I also related the number and recency of brain injuries to measures of psychopathology like depression, anxiety and worry,' she says.

Valera found that of those she interviewed who were in intimate partner violence situations, 75 per cent reported at least one traumatic brain injury. Some reported moderate to severe brain injuries, but most of them reported mild traumatic brain injuries.

'That, in my opinion, is actually pretty shocking and that's a really high number. Especially when you consider the number of women who are in physically abusive relationships.'[269]

These were not just women who were in shelters. That accounted for about half of the women she studied. The other half were still at home.

'Even worse,' she continues, 'is that about 50 per cent, so half of these women, sustained repetitive mild traumatic brain injuries. For a handful of them, it may have been two or three or four or six times. And two or three, maybe not so bad. Anything above that, I'm gonna be more concerned about. And then a lot of them, I just put it in the category of, I think, greater than 20, greater than 25, greater than 30.'

And then there would be those who told her, 'Well, I can't really give you a number. It's too many to count.'

It could have been a couple times a week for several years, or a couple times a month for two years, or something like that.

'So, at that point, you just sort of say, "OK, too many to count is the category we'll put them in," she says.

I ask her what is going to help or influence the rate at which somebody recovers from an injury like this?

'There are a number of different factors,' Eve Valera tells me. 'One of them is basically the acute treatment. If you get treatment right away and you're dealing with it, that's going to help quite a bit. The other is, what else is going on? If you have other physical bodily injuries, that's going to tend to slow down your recovery as well.'

Often, these women have other physical bodily injuries. Additionally, they often have high rates of psychopathology – depression, anxiety, PTSD – that tend to slow down their recovery rate or interact with it in various ways. General life stress is another factor that would influence the general recovery rate. As you can imagine, someone who is in a relationship with an abusive partner is more likely to have a lot of general life stress.

'Then there is the social support or the infrastructure,' Valera says. 'Women who are in violent situations are basically living in what some people refer to as like living in a war zone. They don't necessarily even have the support to do the things that they need to do.'[270]

If you are a top athlete, or even in a car crash, you usually have people around trying to help you, giving you a break, being supportive. These women typically don't have any supporting network like that.

'In terms of recovering, they're really going to be at the most negative end of really any individual I can think of, or type of individual that we know anything about,' Valera says.

Even in the short term, these TBI-related symptoms can have real-world consequences for women trying to get help.

These women commonly need support from multiple sources, including police, legal services and medical and counselling professionals. Attention and memory problems, combined with feelings of depression and anxiety, can make it difficult or impossible to figure out who to contact and where to go, and also to schedule visits and remember complex instructions.

Women with brain injuries make very lousy witnesses because, when we think of a footballer who has a suspected brain injury from a sporting event, the first thing asked is usually 'What half are we in?' 'Who's the opposing team?' or 'What's the score?' Those are the basic things they should be able to remember.

If you go up in front of a judge in a domestic violence situation and you don't remember the incident, you don't remember how you got hit or how many times, you're going to seem like a fake, like you're drunk or you don't have it together: you don't make a credible witness.

I wonder how many judges are prepared for a woman who is not only traumatised, but also has a brain injury, and the pieces that she may not be remembering are not because she's trying to fool you or get something over on the judge or the jury, but that she simply doesn't remember because she has a *brain injury*.

That seems like the part that everyone needs to be aware of – from the legal system, to first responders, down to shelter workers – everybody needs to be aware of that cycle on top of the trauma.

An example of this is that it took three failed attempts before I finally had a conversation with Ella, whose experiences opened this chapter. The first she had forgotten to write down, the second she'd taken the wrong number and the third, her mind had blanked out that the interview was going to take place at all.[271] There are more severe consequences for this kind of memory loss. Forgetting to pick children up from school, leaving the oven on, forgetting where they've parked their car, leaving the front doors unlocked.

When we finally speak, Ella tells me that it wasn't a 'date, date' that brought her and her partner together. She makes quotation marks in the air when she tells me this and then immediately apologises for being 'a bit Ross from *Friends*'.

They met through mutual friends at a dinner party; an environment that isn't usually deemed inappropriate or high risk for meeting somebody. It was a safe space among safe people, not that anyone was scanning the room for abusive potential partners – why would they? It was a conversation that led to gentle flirting that led to walks in a local park that quickly became, by Ella's account, 'the most loving relationship' she had ever had.

'The care and attention he put into everything, into me, was like nothing I'd had before. It was like a movie, like my happiness was the only thing that mattered, it was so important to him that I was OK, like the world would stop if I wasn't!'

At first, I sensed the familiar narrative unravelling, how quickly attention turns to possession, how 'checking in' shifts to the more sinister 'checking up', how suddenly there is intense guilt when adoration has mutated into ammunition – 'But, look at everything I've done for you.'

Only this didn't happen with Ella; there was never any of that, she insists, no signs of manipulation or the textbook abusive behaviour we can break down in a bullet-pointed *Cosmopolitan* magazine check-list article titled 'Six Signs You're Being Abused'. But there was PTSD, which remained hidden for the first six months of their relationship.

'Hidden or managed, I'm not sure which,' Ella offers.

The PTSD would manifest in outbursts of violence, almost exclusively blows to Ella's head.

'It was always over quickly. It came from nowhere. Maybe it was a sound or a word or something totally in his head that made him just switch. He always apologised after and cried. He cried a lot and then in-between he was wonderful. He had a great job, was really good at numbers, played a lot of sport, had friends. Nothing that would indicate he was going to explode. And usually, it was fine. But there was one point when it got really bad.'

Ella describes sitting where we are now, watching the kids in the cul-de-sac whizz past on their bikes. She had made bread, sourdough, and although we agree that certain details would have to be changed for her protection, she was adamant I left that one in because of how very normal it made the afternoon seem.

'It's not exactly a sign of what's to come, is it? Making middle-class bread!' she roared.

She'd been having trouble remembering basic things that day: ingredients when she got to the supermarket, the times of phone calls she was supposed to have with her business partner, the name of a song to send to her sister she had heard on BBC 6 Music literally minutes before she'd unlocked her phone to type the text. I now notice the copious amounts of Post-it notes that adorn her fridge and cupboards, reminders of what's inside them, check lists for the day.

'HAVE YOU TURNED THE HOB OFF?' is written on a neon orange square stuck to the frame of the kitchen door.

'I thought I was stressed or just tired, work was ramping up,' she says. 'I guess I was a little withdrawn and it's crazy to think now how normal the violence had become. How it was just part of the relationship, like, "Oh, he's home, we're having dinner," normal, normal, "Oh, he's hit me, he's sad." We make up, finish dinner, go to bed. There were never bruises, so in a strange way, it was like nothing had happened.'

She pauses, lets out a sigh and I notice her hands balled into fists again.

'Only this time he came in and it was different, he went straight for me, always my head, but this time I'm on the floor. He's knocked me to the floor and . . .'

She lets the words linger for a second; her eyes are no longer meeting mine. She leans forward in her chair; her hands are once again at her temples. She flicks her blonde hair over to one side with a sigh, pulling it into curtains so I can see the scar that runs from her ear to the back of her head into her hair line. It's about two inches long.

Ella can't remember shopping lists, her writing and spelling have deteriorated, her memory functions are much lower than that of other women her age – she forgets things almost instantly.

Sometimes she gets dizzy, her words get mixed up. If she doesn't write things down, she'll never remember them. She has low moods, depression, anxiety, PTSD.

'So, it's not just the pain that I'm left with,' she says. 'It's all of this.'

She gestures to the Post-it notes, her eyes tracing them around the room. I follow her gaze. It was Jude Gibbs that wrote, 'Grief does not demand pity, it requests acknowledgement.'[272]

We sit very quietly, taking it all in. So often we are told that trauma does not define us and yet it's hard to believe that, sitting here now, surrounded by those little neon squares that Ella has come to rely on. The narrative that women are strong and they come through is one I have long championed, but it does women like Ella a disservice. She survived, that much is true, but there are some things that she can never come back from, that have altered life forever. This is what she is left with.

★★★

'There are so many differences between these women and what we know about in terms of traumatic brain injury, which is mostly conducted on all men in somewhat different situations,' Dr Eve Valera observes. 'The idea that someone says, "Well, there's already a study out there, what else do you need to do? How are you advancing the field if you do more work?"'

But the work hasn't been done on this population. Eve Valera thinks some of it's due to misogyny.

'Just a bit!' I laugh.

We only have to look at the #MeToo movement to know that bad things have been happening to women for a very long time and people don't care.

'I think that the idea of domestic violence and intimate partner violence is something people don't want to recognise and accept that that's going on. It's going on right underneath our noses all the time,' she says. 'Now, I'm not saying one in three women are necessarily sustaining repetitive amounts of traumatic brain injuries, but that's still a humongous segment of the population who's sustaining physical or sexual partner violence.'

From her studies, she knows that the rate is high of at least single brain injuries, and repetitive brain injuries are not far behind.

'To me, it's a huge problem that is somehow overlooked. People don't want to admit to it. It's OK if it happens in other countries. Yeah, we know that happens there, but admitting it happens here in the Western world?' She sighs. 'People I know and love will look at my studies and be like, "Are you kidding me? This really happens to people? Seriously?"'

I wonder about CTE, if that even comes into the equation here.

'There are instances of women having things, problems that you would expect to see in substantially older women. That has a feel and a sound of something CTE-like to me,' she responds. 'Will it be the same as what we see in the recorded cases of the football players where they either commit suicide or they are dementing really early, or becoming volatile and hostile and doing really crazy things, to speak loosely? I don't know because we just have not assessed that yet.'[273]

In 2018, in the first study of its kind, the Disabilities Trust provided a dedicated service to support the identification and rehabilitation of female offenders with a history of brain injury in a women's prison, HMP/YOI Drake Hall in London. Comprising staff training, the screening of prisoners and provision of one-to-one support, through a Brain Injury Linkworker (BIL), the service was offered between 2016 and 2018 and the final report included the findings from an independent evaluation of the service conducted by Royal Holloway, University of London.[274]

Despite being a minority within the criminal justice system (CJS), women are some of the most vulnerable prisoners, with behavioural and emotional difficulties. It was thought that a significant number of them were struggling with the consequences of undiagnosed brain injuries. Women in prison are five times more likely to self-harm than men, half are struggling with depression and almost half have made suicide attempts.[275]

Despite only representing 5 per cent of the prison population, women make up a quarter of first-time offenders. Two-thirds were mothers to children under 18 years old, with two-fifths of women claiming that their offending had been driven by the 'need to support their children'.

The Disabilities Trust recognised that while many of the milder symptoms of brain injuries can be 'masked', they nevertheless cause behaviours that can be perceived as 'challenging' and 'difficult' by the CJS. These included: frequently missed appointments, seen as the individual being avoidant or irresponsible, which might be due to poor memory as a result of a brain injury; repeating the same thing over and over again, potentially seen as the individual being rude, but also might be down to poor self-awareness; saying they will do something and never getting around to it, which may be seen as the individual being manipulative or lazy when this may in fact be due to poor initiation as caused by a brain injury.[276]

Previous research from the Ministry of Justice Female Offender Strategy has shown that a significant number of female offenders experience chaotic lifestyles with histories of poor mental health, alcohol and drug misuse. Approximately half report having been victims of physical, sexual or domestic abuse, which are essential factors in understanding an individual's vulnerability to engaging in offending behaviour.[277]

Compared to male offenders, there is limited research investigating the prevalence and impact of brain injuries among female offenders. The Disabilities Trust found that within HMP/YOI Drake Hall, of the 173 female offenders screened, 64 per cent reported a history indicative of a brain injury and of those,

96 per cent reported a history indicative of a traumatic brain injury. There is currently no mandatory routine screening for brain injury, basic awareness training for staff or dedicated brain injury support within UK prisons, despite the fact that behavioural and cognitive consequences of brain injury may have a huge impact on reoffending behaviour and difficulty with engaging in offence-focused rehabilitation programmes. Official figures show that 70 per cent of women reoffend after a year.[278]

How many other people might be out there who can't quite find the right doctor but who aren't quite sure what to do with themselves? How do they find the help?

This was drawn into sharp focus in January 2021 with the execution of Lisa Montgomery, who received a lethal injection at a prison in Terre Haute, Indiana, after a last-minute stay of execution was lifted by the US Supreme Court.[279]

Her defence team believe that at the time of her crime, Montgomery was psychotic and out of touch with reality, an opinion that had been supported by 41 former and current lawyers, as well as human rights groups. As a child, she was routinely sexually and physically abused by her stepfather and trafficked by her mother, family members had testified. Both her mother and stepfather have since passed away, without acknowledging the extent of their abuse.

Lawyers argued that she had been born brain-damaged and that the treatment she received at the hands of her stepfather and captors was so violent that it amounted to torture. They said she was too mentally ill to be executed.

According to a court filing made in the US Southern District of Indiana court, judge James Patrick Hanlon granted a stay of execution to allow the court to conduct a hearing to determine whether she was competent to be executed.[280]

However, the Supreme Court overturned the stay of execution and upheld her sentence.[281]

Her crime was proven to be premeditated and utterly violent. She strangled a pregnant woman, 23-year-old Bobbie Jo Stinnett, before cutting out and kidnapping her baby. The 23-year-old woman bled to death but her baby was safely recovered and returned to her family.

Stinnett's brother-in-law, Ace Stinnett, told the *Sun* in an exclusive interview following Montgomery's execution: 'This brings us closure, we're going on with our lives now. Justice has been served. We just wanted it to be over with. Bobbie Jo would be happy.'[282]

Like Aaron Hernandez, Lisa Montgomery was a murderer in spite of her brain damage. Her case is conflicting, but it's clear that the most vulnerable within our society are being excluded, not just from the conversation, but from any steps of progress towards a solution, recovery or even the prevention of such crimes.

***

Sport and domestic abuse have closer connections in terms of brain injury, too. In their study, 'The punch-drunk boxer and the battered wife', Stephen T. Casper and Kelly O'Donnell cite Bob Fitzsimmons, who is considered to this day as having one of the hardest punches in the history of boxing. He was a British professional boxer and World Heavy Weight Champion, who was taken to court in 1895 for the killing of Con Riordan in a sparring match. He was exonerated but later, in 1901, he would be reprimanded by the police again for punching his third wife in the head. They reconciled shortly afterwards.[283]

Casper and O'Donnell go on to make a link from Fitz-simmons to the 1989 police report filed against football player O.J. Simpson for allegedly beating his wife Nicole Brown Simpson and hypothesise that its cause had a physical basis in brain injury,[284] which Richard Schneider and Elizabeth Crosby called in 1973 'dyscontrol syndrome' in the athlete.[285] Simpson has continually denied assaulting his wife. Later in 2016, in an interview with ABC, Dr Bennet Omalu declared that he would bet his medical licence on O.J. Simson having CTE, after identifying the tell-tale signs of its behavioural symptoms, which include explosive, impulsive behaviour, impaired judgement, criminality and even mood disorders in the former American footballer.[286] But it wasn't used in his trial, which saw Simpson infamously acquitted of the murder of his ex-wife Nicole Brown Simpson and Ron Goldman, her friend (which he has also continuously denied).

It was arguably because of his stellar legal team, but also, in part, his status as a celebrated athlete. Even before he stepped into court, on hearing he was wanted for the double murder, he took to the freeways of southern California in his vehicle and was chased down by police, an event televised live to millions. Fans were lining the streets cheering and chanting 'Free O.J.', while others held signs saying, 'Save The Juice,' as he was fondly known, and 'We Love The Juice'.[287] The mood of that day was reported as being 'festive' and predominantly supportive of Simpson, demonstrating the importance of sport and sports celebrities in society.

A decade later, Lakers basketball star Kobe Bryant became the second athlete in a high-profile case, when he was accused of rape. He had checked into the Cordillera Lodge and Spa in Edwards, Colorado ahead of a knee operation at a clinic in nearby Vail. He was met at the front desk by the female concierge and shown to his room. He requested that she return later to give him a private tour of the property. She did, after which he invited her to his room.

While both of their stories align on what happened immediately on entering the room – they kissed – there are two distinct versions of what happened next. The woman told the police that Bryant raped her, and Bryant insisted they had consensual sex, though he told the police he had not explicitly asked for consent. Court documents revealed that following a hospital examination, the woman was found to have bruises on her neck and tears in her vaginal wall. Both her underwear and Bryant's shirt were bloody.

There was a media frenzy surrounding the story and quickly the accuser's reputation was brought into disrepute, digging up details of her sexual and psychiatric history as evidence that she couldn't be trusted. The *New York Times* reported that Bryant's lawyer, Pamela Mackey, said the woman's name in open court six times during one hearing – even though the police and court officials had tried to preserve her anonymity – and asked if her injuries could have been caused 'by having sex with three men in three days'.

Television crews camped outside the home of the accuser's parents, and her name was leaked by the court system three times. She was hounded by the media, threatened by fans and smeared in the print press. At the time it sparked commentary that perpetuated stereotypes about false accusations of rape.

Eventually, the woman stopped cooperating with the investigation and the case was dropped, though it's unclear why.[288] Perhaps she had made it up and it had gone far enough, or perhaps she was a 19-year-old who had her anonymity taken away and was now facing the most hostile of media thrashings in a fight she could never win, pressured by the astute lawyers of a beloved global sports superstar whose legal resources outnumbered hers over a million to one.

Bryant would later publicly apologise to the woman in the press, acknowledging her perspective of their encounter, despite his own firm belief that it was consensual.

'I recognise now that she did not and does not view this incident the same way I did,' he said.[289] But was it in that non-apology way that doesn't take ownership of any wrongdoing, nor communicate any remorse for the person's actions? It's essentially 'I'm sorry you felt that way', implying that the fault lies in her feelings of the situation, not his actions.

Sporting prowess taking precedent over a victim isn't mutually exclusive to the athletes at the top of their game either. In 2012, Steubenville, Ohio, a small city of 19,000 about 40 miles from Pittsburgh, and its high-school football team, Big Red, became the epicentre of a nationwide media storm when allegations of rape emerged. It was a place that held its football team in the highest regard; the sport was like a religion, whose place of worship was the field on a Friday night. Every time Big Red would score, a sculpture of a stallion named Man O' War would send a six-foot-long stream of fire into the night sky over the stadium.

But in August 2012, two star players from the school's football team, Ma'lik Richmond, 16, and Trenton Mays, 17, were accused of raping a 16-year-old girl from a neighbouring town who was too drunk to consent. The case garnered attention nationwide, in part for the role that social media had played in its development. Several individuals publicised the event, using Twitter, YouTube, Instagram and text messages. Video and photo evidence revealed that the girl was sexually assaulted over the course of several hours. It happened at a party in celebration of Trenton and Ma'lik, who had helped propel Big Red to a victory that now saw a championship firmly on the cards.

'Huge party!!! Banger!!!!' Mays had tweeted on the night of 12 August.

There would be several parties that night, and the following morning a 16-year-old girl would wake up naked in a basement, unable to find her shoes or phone, with no memory of the previous night. She would be collected by friends and taken home, telling her mother immediately that she had no idea what happened until the events of the previous evening began to circulate on social media. In some of the images that had been shared, she saw a naked girl lying on a carpet that she realised matched the basement room she had woken up in.

In a photograph posted on Instagram by Steubenville High football player Cody Saltsman, the victim was shown looking unresponsive, being carried by two teenage boys by her wrists and ankles. Former Steubenville baseball player Michael Nodianos, responding to stories of the event, tweeted, 'Some people deserve to be peed on,' which was retweeted later by several people, including Mays. There was also a tweet exchange with one student with the Twitter handle Kobe Bryant that read 'first degree rape LMAO (laugh my ass off)'.[290] In a 12-minute video later posted to YouTube, Nodianos and others talk about the rapes, with Nodianos joking that 'they raped her quicker than Mike Tyson raped that one girl', and 'they peed on her. That's how you know she's dead, because someone pissed on her'.[291] The video is still online.

The city's police chief begged for witnesses to come forward but received little response. Later, the county prosecutor and the judge in charge of handling crimes by juveniles were excused from the case because they had ties to the football team. Within days, Alexandria Goddard, a Columbus crime blogger, had collected the numerous tweets and messages that had been posted online by the party goers and wrote online that the police and town officials were giving the football players special treatment.

Members of the community were also blaming the girl for her own rape and for the negative light it was now casting on the football team and town. In the 2018 documentary *Roll Red Roll* by Nancy Schwartzman, we see the lead police investigator, J.P. Rigaud, explaining the legal definition of rape to the head football coach in an interview. He had threatened football suspensions for underage drinking, but not for substantiated allegations of sexual assault, which he qualifies with judgements about the decisions the girl had made, rather than the boys. A recording of a local radio host declares over a panning shot of the town that given his knowledge of the football team, the girl likely just didn't want to admit to her parents that she had sex.[292]

Goddard's blog and the town's response garnered attention, prompting women's advocacy groups and the hacker collective Anonymous to get involved.

They hacked the Big Red fan website called RollRedRoll. com and pasted a video on its front page. An ominous Guy Fawkes masked face, its voice-distorted, says, '*You can hide no longer. You have attracted the attention of the hive. We will not sit tightly and watch a group of young men who turn to rape as a game or a sport get the pass because of athletic ability and small-town luck.*'

A Twitter feed called #OpRollRedRoll was started and they demanded an apology by school officials and local authorities, who had allegedly covered up the incident in order to protect the athletes and school's programme.

They also downloaded the emails of the site's operator, making the archive available for download on the Local Leaks website and released the video captured by Nodianos.

It made national news overnight.

Ohio investigators then analysed hundreds of text messages from more than a dozen cell phones and created an almost real-time account of the assault, which read like a graphic, public diary.

'I have no sympathy for whores,' one tweet from the night had read.

'Sloppy,' reads the caption of a blurry photo of a passed-out girl being carried by boys on Instagram.

'She is so raped right now' is heard from a grainy cell phone recording followed by laughter.

Some of the messages that were later read out in court include Mays stating that he had used his fingers to penetrate the girl, whom he referred to in a separate message as 'like a dead body'. In another message, Mays admitted to the girl that he had taken the picture of her lying naked in a basement with what he told her was his semen on her body, not urine as the video had suggested. Though he stated that this was a consensual sex act. The defence attorneys doubled down on this, stating that the girl's judgement wasn't impaired, relying on a strategy concerning levels of drunkenness to prove consent.

A guilty verdict was delivered after five days in court by judge Thomas Lipps who called the crime 'profane' and 'ugly'. In video footage, on hearing their conviction, both boys are in tears. Richmond walks towards the girl's family and says: 'I had not intended to do anything like this. I'm sorry to put you through this,' before breaking down to the point that he is unable to speak. He is embraced by a court officer.

Mays, who most of the evidence surrounds, cries initially, but then stands and walks out more composed, cool almost. He received two years, one for the rape itself and another for distributing the graphic photographs among his peers. Because the girl was a minor, Mays was charged with and convicted of the dissemination of child pornography. Mays's quick recovery to a seemingly unruffled exterior is disturbing. He takes it in his stride as if he's just been sent off the pitch following a foul, either determined not to make it worse or unbothered entirely. He apologises to the victim by name, as well as to her family and the community, not for the act itself but instead for the pictures. 'No pictures should have been sent around, let alone ever taken,' he told them.[293]

Perhaps most telling from all the evidence that was amassed were messages that showed Mays pleading with the girl not to press charges because doing so would damage his football career, seeming to care far more about the sport than the ordeal he had put her through. I can't help but think if it hadn't received so much media attention when Anonymous intervened, thrusting the small town in Ohio into the spotlight, if it hadn't fallen under the gaze of millions of burning eyes across the globe, would there have even been a courtroom for Mays to saunter out of?

And if there was, who would believe a drunken girl over the town's star player?

Months after the incident, Michael Nodianos issued an apology via his attorney Dennis McNamara at a press conference on his behalf saying that his behaviour was disappointing, insensitive and unfortunate: 'After some sober reflection he is ashamed and embarrassed of himself. He's sorry to victims and his family. He was not raised to act in this manner.'

Despite protests within the community, Jefferson County Sheriff Fred Abdalla said that no further suspects would be charged in the rape.[294]

But this wasn't the end of the trial.

The Ohio Attorney General at the time, Mike DeWine, decried 'blurred, stretched and distorted boundaries of right and wrong' by students and grown-ups alike. 'How do you hold kids accountable if you don't hold the adults accountable?' DeWine had asked a press conference.[295] The adults in question included William Rhinaman who was the first to be indicted on three additional felony counts: tampering with evidence, obstruction of justice and perjury, as well as obstructing official business (a second degree misdemeanor). He was the former technology director for Steubenville City Schools and pleaded guilty to obstructing official business, a second-degree misdemeanor, after deleting files from the Steubenville computer network that were relevant to the case. He was sentenced to 90 days of jail, 80 of which were to be suspended upon completion of a year of probation and 40 hours of community service.

The Steubenville Superintendent at the time, Michael McVey, was accused of a third-degree felony count of tampering with evidence, two fifth-degree felony counts of obstructing justice, a first-degree misdemeanor count of falsification and a second-degree misdemeanor count of obstructing official business. He pleaded not guilty and charges were dismissed in exchange for his resignation as superintendent. He was not to seek employment with Steubenville schools in the future.

A volunteer high-school football coach, the principal of Steubenville elementary school, and an assistant wrestling coach and special education teacher were also indicted.

They were placed on administrative leave, though both the wrestling coach and elementary principal were returned to their positions as both employees had 'good work records and presumed innocent until proven guilty'.

The volunteer coach was sentenced to ten days in jail. He was the only adult present at the party attended by both Richmond, Mays and the victim. He was the first adult to be sentenced in the case.

'It's very unfortunate the events that transpired that night, you know, with the girl and everything,' he said in court. Believing he made the 'the right decisions', but 'I didn't make the decisions quick enough'.

He said he learned 'that no matter what, you should always tell the truth'.

He was also ordered to serve 40 hours of community service and pay $1,000 in fines. Two other charges, obstructing official business and contributing to the unruliness or delinquency of a child, were dismissed.

Ohio Attorney General Mike DeWine later dropped the charges against the elementary principal and the wrestling coach in exchange for both to undertake community service volunteering at a rape crisis centre and help develop a sexual-assault awareness programme.

The football coach, Reno Saccoccia, was not indicted despite the court hearing text messages from Mays that allege his complicity in the act. They read:

I got Reno. He took care of it and s*** ain't gonna happen, even if they did take it to court.

In 2012 a change.org petition was started titled 'Steuben-ville Schools: Fire Coach Reno Saccoccia', which gathered 136,000 signatures. Despite this, 2020 marked his fiftieth sea-son of football coaching.[296]

Of all the adults tried in relation to the Stuebenville case, it was the anonymous hacker that got the biggest sentence. Following an FBI raid on his house, he recalled that 'approx-imately 12 FBI SWAT team agents jumped out of the truck, screaming for me to "Get the fuck down!" with M-16 assault rifles and full riot gear, armed, safety off, pointed directly at my head'.[297]

Deric Lostutter was sentenced to two years in federal prison by a judge in Lexington, Kentucky, for conspiring to illegally access a computer without authorisation and lying to an FBI agent. Trenton Mays was also sentenced to serve two years in the State Juvenile System for the rape.

Under the nickname KYAnonymous, Lostutter had formed the KnightSec hacking crew that hacked into the fan website of the Steubenville High School football team together with Noah McHugh, a.k.a. JustBatCat. Lostutter said he didn't do any of the actual hacking himself, noting that McHugh took credit for it in an interview with the *Herald Star*.

Noah McHugh received an eight-month prison sentence after pleading guilty to one count of computer fraud. Court records said McHugh began cooperating with federal prose-cutors in April 2013 and he testified against Lostutter during a grand jury hearing.

A statement issued by the Department of Justice reads that 'Lostutter filmed a video wearing a mask and wrote a manifesto, which were both posted on the website to harass and intimi-date people, and to gain publicity for Lostutter's and McHugh's online identities.' It also states that 'the messages threatened to reveal personal identifying information of Steubenville High School students, and made false claims that the administrator of the fan website was involved in child pornography and directed a "rape crew"'.[298]

Carlton S. Shier, IV, Acting United States Attorney for the Eastern District of Kentucky, said that 'computer hacking and cyber harassment create real victims, causing enormous damage to real people, organisations, and institutions. This type of conduct simply cannot be tolerated and the great work of our FBI partners in this matter validates our ongoing efforts to protect the public from illegal computer intrusions and other cybercrime'.[299]

In an interview with *Mother Jones*, Lostutter said he believed that the FBI investigation was motivated by local officials in Steubenville. 'They want to make an example of me, saying, "You don't fucking come after us. Don't question us,"' he claimed.

Lostutter was sentenced to more time than Richmond, a convicted rapist.

It's a depressing message to send out for men who stick up for women.

Cody Saltsman sued Goddard and the commenters on her blog for defamation, though he eventually dismissed the suit, choosing instead that the blog issue a formal apology.

I deeply regret my actions on the night of August 11, 2012. While I wasn't at the home where the alleged assault took place, there is no doubt that I was wrong to post that picture from an earlier party and tweet those awful comments. Not a moment goes by that I don't wish I would have never posted that picture or tweeted those comments. I want to sincerely apologize to the victim and her family for these actions. I also want to acknowledge the work of several bloggers, especially Ms. Goddard at Prinniefied.com, in their efforts to make sure the full truth about that terrible night eventually comes out. At no time did my family mean to stop anyone from expressing themselves online – we only wanted to correct what we believed were mis statements that appeared on Ms. Goddard's blog. I am glad that we have resolved our differences with Ms. Goddard and that she and her contributors can continue their work.

– Cody Saltsman[300]

On his release it was reported that Ma'lik Richmond returned to Steubenville High School and rejoined the football team, with the blessing of the team's long-time head coach, Reno Saccoccia. 'I feel that we're really not giving him a second chance,' Saccoccia said in an interview with WTVR Channel 6. 'Some may look at it like that. I feel he has earned a second chance. We don't deal in death sentences for juvenile activity and I just feel that he's earned a second chance … It was a horrible crime; it was a horrible crime,' Saccoccia told WTVR. 'Everything the judicial system of Ohio asked him to do, he completed "Everything that the school system asked him to do upon his release, he completed both academically and socially. He was back in school since January, and was suspended from all extracurricular activities for the remainder of the year."'

Steubenville wasn't the only example where the immediate concern in a sex assault wasn't for the survivor's future, but the perpetrators'. In 2015, former Stanford University swimmer Brock Turner was charged with sexually assaulting an unconscious woman on campus. The judge, Aaron Persky, a Stanford alumnus, announced a sentence of only six months in jail – stating that positive character references and lack of a criminal record had persuaded him to be more lenient. Prison would have a 'severe impact on him', he said of Turner.[301]

This was despite the fact that two witnesses saw Turner 'thrusting' on top of the motionless woman, and intervened and held him until police arrived, and a jury ultimately convicted him of assault with intent to rape an intoxicated woman, and sexually penetrating an intoxicated and unconscious person with a foreign object. The leniency of the sentence caused outcry, made worse by Turner's father who declared his son was paying a 'steep price' for '20 minutes of action'. Boys will be boys, after all.

The judge was accused of making women at Stanford and across California less safe and perpetuating a message that women and girls are on their own, while the prevailing message to potential perpetrators was 'you will be protected'.

Social media became enraged, with many accounts quoting the survivor's impact statement, which was released by the district attorney's office and published in full by online platform *Buzzfeed*.

'I thought there's no way this is going to trial; there were witnesses, there was dirt in my body, he ran but was caught . . . Instead, I was told he hired a powerful attorney, expert witnesses, private investigators . . . That he was going to go to any length to convince the world he had simply been confused.'

She said: 'I was pummelled with narrowed, pointed questions that dissected my personal life, love life, past life, family life – inane questions, accumulating trivial details to try and find an excuse for this guy who had me half naked before even bothering to ask for my name.'[302]

Turner was sentenced to six months and released after serving three, and remains on the sex offenders' register. The survivor provided her statement in full to *BuzzFeed News* which quickly went viral and later, in 2019, she allowed her name, Chanel Miller, to be made public and released her memoir, *Know My Name*.

'Your damage was concrete; stripped of titles, degrees, enrolment,' she wrote. 'My damage was internal, unseen, I carry it with me.'[303]

I have thought about consent a lot throughout this investigation. Who is protected and who isn't? And in whose hands does the power to protect lie?

***

We know that men's violence against women and girls has become a global pandemic. The *Guardian* reported in February 2020 that the latest UK Femicide Census shows that, despite more than 50 years of feminist campaigning against male violence, the number of women and girls dying at the hands of men is increasing.[304]

In London, domestic violence has risen by 63 per cent in the last seven years and these are just the cases that we know about; on average, domestic abuse victims will have been assaulted 35 times before reporting it to the police.

But while our awareness has grown, any prevalence of CTE in these situations remains to be seen. Aside from the cases I have mentioned, there have not been any systematic studies evaluating CTE in women.

There was something that kept coming up in my conversations with Dawn Astle, with Peter Robinson, with the various ex-players and researchers I'd spoken to – that the athletes know the risk, that anyone stepping back into the ring has an expectation of injury. But what if that ring is your home? Your opponent your partner?

Women are so often asked the tone-deaf question, 'Why don't you just leave?'

Sometimes it's because they can't for the life of them figure out how, or that they have become dependent on a partner because they can't function alone with children, or that their departure poses an even greater threat to their lives and the lives of their children than staying and enduring more violence.

'There are people out there who will say, "Well, if it's so bad, why don't they just get out? It's kind of your own fault if you don't leave,"' Eve Valera says, shaking her head. 'This idea that if you choose to stay in that relationship, then you['ve] got to take your lumps and bumps. Which is just a horrible, horrible, horrible response.'[305]

F.K.A. Twigs said it best in an interview she gave to British broadcaster Louis Theroux, following the accusations of abuse that she made public against former partner Shia LaBeouf, which the actor vehemently denies: 'The question should really be to the abuser: ask them why are you holding someone hostage with abuse?'[306]

***

Katherine Snedaker is the founder of PINK Concussions, the first non-profit organisation focused on female brain injury, which looks at brain injury from several mechanisms including domestic violence, military service and sports injury. I met Katherine in New York. She is well acquainted with Dr Eve Valera and almost all of the people who've contributed their expertise to this book. It's a small world once you've been let through the doors.

When the foundation began, Snedaker had wanted to look at sport, domestic violence and the military, but was told 'by very smart people', she says, that it was a bad idea. She was told to pick just one. 'But I was like, how can you break those apart?!'[307]

Snedaker believes that unless you combine the research, you will never get a whole picture – and that makes sense because all of these groups include women who are at risk of being hit repeatedly and in the same way. Just as we train sports coaches and parents to recognise that an injury could be a possible brain injury, PINK Concussions is trying to work with domestic violence shelters to give them the same base knowledge.

There are few women with brain injuries that we know of and a smaller network of women to talk to. Katherine, a breast cancer survivor, compares the experience of recovery.

'When you're going through cancer there are so many women out there that you're networked through, from friends and family, from church and work. When you have a brain injury – silence, crickets. No one to connect to.'

There's more male brain injury out there, that much is true, I say.

'[I]t's also an excuse,' Katherine says. 'There are more men because they've studied men and male animals in the research rather than female. But if you look at what a woman experiences, it's different to men.'

On top of this, she suggests that most women will likely only know other males who are suffering from concussion, which is also problematic.

'So, say I've been diagnosed with concussion. I'm three weeks out. I'll go talk to the three men I know that had a concussion, and they'll say, "Oh yeah, we were better in a week." So, now she's starting to doubt herself. "Why am I not better?

Is there something wrong with me? Am I faking it? Maybe I'm not doing it right or I'm weak.'"

The difference, she thinks, is the expectation that women need to be given more of a runway for their recovery, and have their employers, their family, their spouses, their parents, their teachers say, 'Hey, this might take more time than you're used to seeing it take.' And the more you support the person and the more you say, 'Hey, we're here for you,' then they don't have the stress of being isolated and thinking something is wrong with them.

Since its inception, PINK Concussions has led campaigns that have resulted in hundreds of women signing over their brains for scientific research. Among these women are sporting stars, including World Cup winner Brandi Chastain, who was the second national team member to donate her brain, after American soccer player and president of the American Soccer Federation, Cindy Parlow Cone.

Parlow Cone played from the time she could walk until she retired after the 2004 Olympics. She won two Olympic gold medals. Up until 2004, she had suffered two diagnosed concussions and then several other concussions where she had seen stars after heading the ball. She didn't think much of them because, at the time, concussions weren't really part of the discussion. But in 2004, as she was training for the Olympics, she was having headaches pretty much every day and severe jaw pain and couldn't figure out why she couldn't get fit. She was tired all the time, sleeping about 15 hours, but she never correlated it back to the concussions that she suffered because all the doctors had told her she was fine.

'As an athlete, when you hear that from a doctor . . . you can go back and play – that's all you need to hear – and so I thought there was something like maybe I took too much time off or I wasn't training the right way,' she said.[308]

She was always a player. Always a lover of not just the game but also the training, and all of a sudden she wasn't looking forward to any of it anymore. Some days she didn't want to go and would have to drag herself there. She just wanted to push through, to get through 2004 with the Olympics. She did, even taking gold. But then afterwards, she decided that it was time to take a break from the sport and try to get healthy.

'Keep in mind my concussions were 15 years ago,' she says. 'We didn't really have the understanding of concussions that we do today and so I thought pushing through my symptoms and trying to be tough was the way to go about it. But we know differently now and if I had to do it all over, obviously I would have sat out and fully recovered until all of my symptoms went away and then gradually got back into the sport. To this day, I still have the same symptoms that I did when I initially had my concussions in 2001 and 2003 and they affect my everyday life.'[309]

She publicly argued against heading in youth soccer because of the impact that heading a football has had on her life and in November 2015, US Soccer announced stricter standards for players under 14.

She isn't the only member of the revered US World Cup team to speak about concussion though. Ever since she was seven years old, Brianna Scurry had wanted to be an Olympian. She would go on to find her way to the podium not once but twice, winning gold both times. She had a prolific career in goal, playing at international level from 2008. On 25 April 2010, however, her life changed forever when during a match, Scurry hit the side of her head on an opposing player's knee. Since the incident occurred, she has had dizziness, imbalance, memory loss, difficulty sleeping, sensitivity to light, sound and movement. She's scared.

'Granted I was 30 years old and I had already had a fantastic career. But even at 30 I wasn't quite ready to be done yet,' she says.[310]

According to a 2011 study in the *American Journal of Sports Medicine*, in high-school sports that have similar rules for boys and girls, namely football or soccer, girls get concussions at twice the rate as boys. Another study found that among all collegiate athletes, female soccer players had the highest overall concussion rates.[311]

Doctors initially estimated that Brianna would need a few days to recover, as most people who suffer concussions do. When her symptoms persisted, they revised that estimate to two weeks. Then 60 days. Then indefinitely. In that time, she has undergone several months of therapy where doctors didn't quite know what was wrong with her, of subjective testing, in which doctor after doctor would tell her, month after month, year after year, that she should be fine. That she *should* be better. She became depressed, she had anxiety.

'I was not myself. I was suicidal. And that was the hardest three or four years of my life,' she says. It wasn't until 2013 that she was finally diagnosed with post-concussive syndrome, which can last for weeks, months or years.

'Thank goodness I found a doctor who could diagnose me properly. I ended up having his surgery ironically at Georgetown. Bilateral occipital nerve surgery. And it was a huge success for me. Two months after that I started my therapy with my balance and my cognitive issues. And a year later I was finally fired, as I like to say, by my doctor in October 2014.' This was four years after the initial incident.

I can't help but think, if a two-time gold-medal-winning Olympian with access to the best doctors struggled for years to find the right doctor, the right treatment, what chance would a female survivor of domestic abuse have? So many people are out there who might not be able to find the right doctor, who aren't even sure how to go about it, what to do with themselves. What do these women do? The system is failing them.

'It's a battleground.'

— Dr Robert Cantu

Chapter Nine

A Delicate Game

January 2022 marked 11 years since the death of 14-year-old Benjamin Robinson from injuries sustained while playing school rugby. While his case has been deemed 'rare' and, indeed, an 'accident', his mother, Karen, and father, Peter, have to live with the decisions made during their son's rugby game for the rest of their lives. Lives that no longer include their son.

When news broke of Benjamin's death in the 'sin bin' at Twickenham stadium – the café for staff and officials – Professor Adam J. White, who was in the room, had shrugged it off. 'He could have just as easily died in a car crash,' he said. He was then a top coach for the Rugby Football Union (RFU) – 'It's just a fluke accident,' he had rationalised.[312] His stance is very different now, the opposite in fact, as he has dedicated his career to advocating for safety in the sport.

Over a decade later and the discourse around brain injury in rugby and UK football has been building, with a particular focus on youth participation. The humanity of the problem has seemingly shrunk further and further away, however, with an increasing number of articles being written by those with no expertise in brain trauma, brain health or neurology, including the headmaster of the school where rugby was invented, saying the proposed banning of tackling 'would kill the sport'.[313]

But the families, left picking up the pieces are being forgotten, or worse, trolled, because of their efforts to reform the sports that have taken away their children, and in their bid to save other people from the same unnecessary fate.

On 18 December 2020, an open letter, written by Dr Adam J. White, Professor Allyson Pollock, Professor Eric Anderson and Graham Kirkwood was released to address the removal of the tackle in school rugby.[314] They are four among a host of people who have done stacks of work trying to advocate for keeping children safe and preventing them from suffering concussions. This included recent research funded and conducted by the RFU that has highlighted the lack of evidence for any discernible physical health benefits from full-contact rugby union compared with non-contact codes of rugby, such as touch rugby. This RFU scoping exercise concluded that: 'Across the spectrum of participation, contact rugby union has high injury and concussion incidence rates relative to other sports.'[315]

In 2012, Dr Robert Cantu wrote a book, *Concussion and Our Kids*,[316] advocating that there should be no tackling in American football until high school, that kids should play flag or touch, but not tackle, that there be no heading in soccer until the age of 14 in high school and that there be no full-body checking in ice hockey until high school.

He has a point.

Like the NFL, the National Hockey League also faced controversy in the form of a lawsuit first filed in 2013 by over 300 retired players who accused it of failing to protect them from head injuries or warning them of the risks involved with playing. It's the same story again and again. The settlement tentatively included free neuropsychological tests, up to $75,000 for medical treatment, a potential cash payment of about $20,000 a player and the establishment of a Common Good Fund to help other players in need, and was finally agreed, although in 2020, it reared an uglier head when the National Hockey League was embroiled in a legal fight with insurance companies that refused to pay most of the costs related to the league's years-long concussion lawsuit and the settlement the league reached with retired players.[317] It's never ending, it seems, and no sport is exempt.

'But there's been retaliation. And I get it,' Dr Cantu says.

I remark that he's being incredibly understanding given everything that has happened and is happening still.

'But I mean, if I'm going to stick my neck out, I can fully understand the other side has got every right to try to chop it off!' He laughs. I instantly like him. He speaks slowly and in a measured way. He is self-assured but still warm – a real expert and good advocate, I think.

'But I believe that strongly, and I believe that the research data that I'm aware of supports it. And that's why I'm willing to put my chin out there, so to speak,' he explains.[318]

It's a bit easier for Dr Cantu than for others, something he readily admits. '[A]lthough I'm affiliated, you know, as a clinical professor at Boston University and neurosurgery and neurology, some individuals are connected to tertiary institutions where they are not encouraged to be a part of controversy.

You know what I'm trying to say?' he asks me with a slight smile.[319] I do.

'And I've fortunately never been muzzled by the organisations that we have been a part of. And that's been fortunate for me. Also, it's true as a neurosurgeon that I didn't make my money to feed my family on research. I made it on practising medicine and neurosurgery and therefore I didn't have to worry about whether I was, you know, incurring the wrath of anybody or the people that might be peer reviewing a research grant I was submitting, or an institution may not fund me because they didn't like the results I'd found.'

I ask if this has happened.

'Well, it's in the United States. Probably one of the more high-profile situations is that Bob Stern, one of the co-founders of the CTE Centre, BU with Ann [McKee], and I were in line to receive the $16-million grant from the National Institutes of Health, and that grant was going to be funded by the National Football League. Only, they didn't like who the committee had decided should receive the grant, meaning Bob and his group.'

The NFL pulled the money, or at least that's what's been widely written.[320]

'Fortunately, they found other funding from other places. That study is now in its third year of a seven-year run,' he says.

It's the summer of 2020, and the day before our call, Dr Robert Cantu was on a six-and-a-half-hour call as part of his role as senior adviser to the NFL. The presentation was on the subject of repetitive head trauma.

'They basically found that there wasn't a problem with repetitive head injury,' Cantu says, detached from any emotion. 'Which, of course, the National Football League would have loved to hear.' I sense the hint of a smile.

The report allegedly concluded that no correlation was found between those playing collision sports before the age of 12 and having a higher change in behavioural, cognitive or mood patterns later in life.

'To its credit, the National Football League has put forward over a million dollars to study better protecting against head injury. It's also put forward $40 million directly in terms of studying head injury and the effects of head injury,' Dr Cantu says. 'But it feels like they've kind of picked or chosen who they would like to receive their funds – who have gone down the route of only publishing what, you know, is going to be favourable.'[321]

'Which isn't necessarily completely truthful, is it?' I ask.

'Well, I don't want to say. It is what it is,' Dr Cantu responds diplomatically. 'And all I can say is that, to me, [studies] need to be done by people who have been selected in a non-biased way, completely independently evaluated.' When I put this claim to the NFL, they did not respond.

There are four publications from the Boston group that Cantu and Chris Nowinski co-founded back in 2007, with Bob Stern and Ann McKee. The group has four different publications and different data sets but all the findings are the same. That is, if you start playing American football before the age of 12 and you play it through high school and college and professionally, you're going to have a greater statistical chance of developing cognitive, behavioural and mood problems than if you started playing football at a later age and therefore had less exposure.

Each of those tests were carried out with detailed neuropsychological testing, cognitive testing, mood testing of depression, anxiety and impulsivity, and testing for behavioural regulation in individuals.

'But there is a stark difference between simply asking somebody how they're doing versus giving them a test to see how they're actually doing,' Cantu says. 'Because when you do give people detailed neuropsychological tests, sometimes you find that they say they're doing fine and they're actually doing very poorly. And you even find the opposite. You find people saying, "I'm doing terribly," but they actually do pretty well on the tests. So, you can't rely on what somebody tells you.'

Cantu concludes that although it sounds like there is a lot of detail in the surveys that were done (there's that diplomacy again), it's still incredibly frustrating.

'The battle goes on and on,' he says, with a gentle shrug. 'And unfortunately, there are millions and millions of dollars to be gleaned for research. So, a researcher would always like to say, "We need more study because that means we can get more money for more funding and that's how we survive." So, there are a lot of cross-incentives to coming up with the right answers. And it's very unfortunate that we don't have a system where the data is able to be looked at by everybody.'

I ask him if he called it out yesterday when he spoke with the NFL – did he direct them to the papers that had come from his centre? He did, and quickly confirms that he pointed them in that direction. They agreed with him that the surveys were not as scientifically accurate as actually studying people and having them do detailed tests, but Cantu thinks that information will be drowned out in a few weeks. The paper itself, or a quote from the NFL surrounding it, has yet to emerge.

Dr Cantu is almost annoyingly fair in our conversation – he doesn't need to discredit or bad mouth anybody; he is confident in his work but also the data and the research. I suggest that perhaps the sporting bodies hold information back, that they eke out a bit if it's necessary, that I'm not sure if this is a decision made on morals or money anymore.

'Well, it's because of a variety of things,' he says. 'First, maybe their background is different and they honestly don't believe the same way I believe. But I think that what is unfortunate is that the organisations that they're a part of, that fund their means, have a vested interest in there not being a connection between repetitive head injury in later-life issues.'

What keeps him going is that he believes he is doing the right thing. 'What the research that we've done personally, and been exposed to, and are a part of [shows] is that repetitive head trauma has consequences for a lot of people later in life if they've had too much of it and the consequences fall into baskets of cognitive behavioural problems. And you don't have to have CTE to have those problems. Even without CTE, just too much head trauma could lead to cognitive impairments or mood disruption.'

It is now well established that young players under the age of 18 are particularly vulnerable to concussive injuries because of the maturing and the dynamic neurophysiological state of the adolescent brain. Despite this, the group undertook a 2018 survey of a sample of 288 state secondary schools and found that 76 per cent of boys in English state-funded secondary schools are required by their school to participate in contact rugby in PE lessons as part of the curriculum, and that most heads of PE perceive contact rugby to be the highest-risk activity.

A study published in 2018 by the Royal Society of Medicine revealed almost 50 per cent of sport-injury-related trips to A&E involve children and adolescents, and that 14-year-old boys and 12-year-old girls were the most at risk of sports injuries. Researchers from Newcastle University and Oxford

University NHS Trust investigated 11,676 A&E visits for sports injuries, and found 10- to 14-year-olds were most likely to be injured, followed closely by the 15-to-19-years age group. The main sports involved in boys requiring hospital treatment were football, rugby union and rugby league.[322]

It feels like the uncertainties and the push for concrete evidence surrounding CTE have been such a point of focus throughout history that we have lost sight of the bigger picture. That even if it isn't CTE, repetitive head trauma can cause a multitude of problems in both adults and children. It's a reality that has been incredibly challenging to those that are part of major sport federations, where such trauma is seen as part and parcel of the activity or sport.

The proposed ban on children's tackling and heading received mixed responses, particularly from the public, as witnessed across social media. The 280-character tirade from a troll exudes the message that they would rather be sorry than safe. Grieving parents have been deemed 'too emotionally attached' or accused of 'scaremongering' – their voices often simply cannot cut through the noise.

'You're making the sport soft', 'let them learn how to be men' and 'you're ruining the game' are some of the arguments that have circulated against the ban.

Professor Allyson Pollock has been writing about the dangers of tackling for over 15 years. The first line of her book, *Tackling Rugby: What Every Parent Should Know*, states: 'Today in the United Kingdom it is almost impossible to have a rational conversation about the risks of rugby without provoking shrill cries about the nanny state.'[323]

Pollock has been criticised immensely by the public and the press who felt she had no business in rugby. It's true, she had no business in rugby, no investments or pay cheque that ran through a club or federation – so she was free to sing.

Reviewers in favour of tackling have scorned her for being too close to the 'story', as she responded to rugby's violence as a direct result of two personal experiences – one that saw her good friend and fellow junior doctor left paralysed, and the other involving her own son.

The word 'story' implies something fictitious or dramatised, yet Pollock is a health-care professor and one of the four writers of the 2020 open letter previously mentioned, along with Adam J. White, advocating for better safety in sports. Her son suffered serious injury on three occasions before the age of 16: a broken nose, a fractured leg and a fractured cheekbone with concussion. In 2014, she said, 'Rugby union in schools must distinguish itself from the *very brutal* game practised by the professionals.' Until her son was injured, like every other parent, Pollock says she trusted the school and the authorities to look after him and not expose him to the risk of serious harm. Until she saw it for herself: her son's face smashed in and a cheekbone badly broken during a game.

'I was shocked to the core by his deformed face: his shattered cheek, his eye drooping down and his inability to eat or drink anything but liquids through a straw. Much later, he would tell me that this third injury was a life-changing event that shook his confidence and affected his academic progress and other activities,' she wrote in an *Independent* article in 2014 titled 'Is rugby still too dangerous to play?'

Her language, though emotive, is grounded in science and years of dedicated research. But it's been suggested that she is pushing her own agenda, that she is 'too close' because of her personal experience, that she is being over-protective or 'wrapping children in cotton wool'.

I think of Karen at the side of the pitch in January 2011 as Benjamin lay on the ground for 90 seconds.

It's difficult for me to fully comprehend: parents that once stood at the side of a pitch now stand by the side of a grave, but then again, how could anyone that hadn't been through it themselves truly understand? You can argue with the science, which is very much still in its infancy. You can argue with sport – either for or against it; there are parties on both sides of that fence – but you cannot argue with a bereaved parent. There is no grey area in losing a child as a direct result of the sport they played. Especially if the injuries sustained were preventable.

The thought sits heavily on my chest, because there are others. There are parents all over the world burying their children. I couldn't have anticipated that an investigation into CTE would bring me here, but here I am. Karen and Peter aren't alone.

In the US, more than 3.5 million children aged 14 and younger get hurt annually playing sports or participating in recreational activities.[324] Although death from a sports injury is rare, the leading cause of death from a sports-related injury is a brain injury, with sports and recreational activities contributing to approximately 21 per cent of all traumatic brain injuries among American children.[325]

'There is no justifiable reason whatsoever that a child under the age of 18 in the developed world in Europe, should engage in high-impact contact sports like football, ice hockey, rugby, mixed martial arts, boxing, wrestling!' an impassioned

Dr Bennet Omalu told me.[326] But while sports bodies accept that there is a potential link, they claim more evidence is needed before definitive action is taken, which could mean players potentially being exposed to years of harm until a decision is made.

Studies have shown us that if you play American football, even for just one season, you could suffer permanent brain damage; the more seasons you play the greater the likelihood of progressive brain damage becomes.[327] 'Studies have also shown that in one game of American football, a child receives between 50 to 60 violent blows to their head – and some of those blows are equivalent to a car travelling at a rate of 30 miles an hour, running into a brick wall,' Omalu says.[328]

The Concussion Legacy Foundation in Boston released a video that featured a number of children attempting to spell the word 'concussion' and then describe what it is. It's a telling watch – amusing when they get it so wrong but a stark reminder that they are not aware of the consequences.

'Let that child, growing up to become an adult, reach the age of consent and then make up his mind whether he wants to play or not play,' Dr Bennet Omalu says. 'When we discovered that cigarette smoking was dangerous what did we do? We did not ban cigarette smoking. We protected our children from cigarette smoking. So, if you wouldn't give a child a cigarette to smoke . . . [and] we wouldn't give a glass of fine cognac to a child to drink, why would we then place a helmet on the head of each child and send him to a field on a Saturday morning to intentionally slam his head on the heads of other children and suffer brain damage? Why?'[329]

I wonder how many of those emailing and tweeting bereaved parents, researchers and neuroscientists have ever truly thought about that 'why'. Those people who so regularly and aggressively cite the rise of obesity in young people as a much graver problem to solve than brain trauma, excusing the violence of the game. I have seen emails that question where else boys will get their masculinity from if the game is altered for safety. Emails that draw on the sender's seminal years of playing private-school rugby and how essential it was to their own development as a man. I would argue that that, too, is an emotional attachment to a game. A game that has since mutated tenfold while academic papers are scrutinised and belittled. I'm curious as to what the purpose of those papers would be if not to protect, who they are intended to serve other than the players on the pitch or the ones still to come, why scientists would endeavour to 'destroy' a sport with false information or fear mongering and risk discrediting decades of work and why any parent would relive their grief over and over again if they didn't believe it might just save another life.

But if there's anything I've learnt by now, it's that the human brain is complex.

★★★

It is early in the evening when I speak to John Gaal, Sr. The inky sky hangs heavy like velvet, its hem dipped in golds and purples like a bruise. The night is still, nothing breathes; it's cold but comforting somehow. Safe and quiet.

'Do you know St Louis?' John asks me and I instantly regret selecting the second of the two references that I have – the musical and the character 'Louise from St Louis' played by Jennifer Hudson in the first *Sex and the City* movie. He hasn't seen it and I don't have much to say on it either, but it seems to crack the tension a little.

John Sr and his wife, Mary, live in St Louis, Missouri, and have four children. Their eldest son, John Jr, or Little John as he was fondly known, adored sport like his father but was torn between soccer and American football – his high school would only allow him to choose one, although this didn't deter him. At school he would play American football but outside of that he played in an organised church soccer league during the weekends for his Catholic grade school parish team.

His love of soccer came from his father. In his early years, John Sr loved to play the game. It was part of his life at elementary school. He continued to play as a young adult, and this included one year while in college.

'For the first 28 years of my life, soccer was part of it and it was a good, worldly experience,' John Sr tells me, 'and so when my children were old enough to begin, you know, walking around, they started to learn how to dribble. And I took pride in getting every one of my kids to learn how to use both feet! Because in the USA, a lot of times people are perfectionists with one foot, but not very good with the other. So, my kids were just as good with the left foot as they were with the right-foot, even though they were all dominant right-foot players!'

John Jr was also on the track and field team during the spring months. He competed in four events, the four by two hundred, the four by one hundred sprints, as well as high jump and pole vaulting. He was a versatile athlete – one I've seen captured in high-school movies – blond hair, broad shoulders and a big smile.

'Oh yeah,' John Sr says. 'He just had tremendous upper-body strength and he was as fast as lightning. Little John had an incredible vertical leap standing still. He could easily jump three feet in the air. No, you know what?' he corrects himself mid-flow. '*One metre* in the air. Wow!' he exclaims. 'Just standing still without any running start or anything like that!'

At the end of his second year of high school, John Jr decided he wanted to go to a different school closer to where the family lived. He chose John F. Kennedy Catholic High and as he was about to enter the fall of 2009, the first semester of his third year, he went to his father for some advice. He wondered, since the new school was much smaller than the school he had left, whether they would allow him to play American football and soccer in the same season.

'And I said, "Well, there's only one way you could find out – go and ask,"' John Sr says. John Jr wrote to the athletic director of his school who said as long as he made both coaches aware of what he had chosen as his primary sport, he had his blessing to do both.

'In fact, I told him that, while he was at it, ask for your little brother too. In the back of my mind all I could think about was how great it would be to see both my boys playing on the same varsity teams together.'

John Jr picked American football as his primary sport. While Jake, his little brother, chose soccer as his primary sport.

'And that was life-changing. I mean, I could see change in those first six weeks. His whole demeanour transformed for the better,' John Sr says. 'I mean, he was so happy, so happy!' His son was also busy: if he wasn't at soccer practice it was American football; if it wasn't a football game, it was a soccer game.

I asked John Sr what it was like to watch his son play.

'That field was his stage,' he says proudly. 'His first game on his home field and his last game on his home field were historical, and it was because of him.'

I asked him to take me through those matches. The first was an American football match, one of two that made memories. Certainly, the matches that announced to the world that John Jr had arrived. He played both ways as a running back and safety. Players usually specialise in offence or defence; playing both ways means that John was chosen to do both. The primary roles of a running back are to receive handoffs from the quarterback, to rush the ball, to line up as a receiver to catch the ball, and to block. Safeties are the last line of defence; they are expected to be reliable tacklers, and many safeties rank among the hardest hitters in football. They were positions that complemented John's athleticism, his speed, his strength, as well as his sheer determination.

The match was against his father's old school. John Jr's school hadn't won a football game for three years and they hadn't beaten his father's old school for seven. It was getting late in a very close game. John Sr jumps straight in to setting the scene, half proud parent, half roaring commentator, taking me through the match play by play.

It was the final few minutes of the game and the intensity was rising.

'And the other team was in our red zone, and you know red is seen as a warning colour for the defence! They were 20 yards out from our goal line with the possibility of winning very late in the game. And John, being a safety, sometimes you've got to gamble! And he gambled and he tipped the ball and, you know, knocked it away from one player, which would have scored a touchdown. But unfortunately, it went into someone else's hands and they scored! And so, you know, now here's the new kid that just screwed everything up and you could hear the parents grumbling around me. And actually, a friend of mine who I work with said to me, "I don't think John should have gambled like that." I said, "Don't worry about it. There's plenty of time left!"'

There was only about a minute and a half left. John picks up his pace once more.

'And I told him, I said, "You know, he's like his old man. He is so pissed off right now, I would hate to be the person who's going to get hit!" And lo and behold, they kick off to us because they just scored and they're ahead and we fumble.'

A fumble describes when a player who has possession and control of the ball loses it before being tackled, scoring or going out of bounds. By rule, it is any act other than passing, kicking, punting or successful handling that results in loss of the ball's possession by a player.

'So, they take the ball over and then march it down into our red zone again!'

There was now half a minute left. John Sr doesn't miss a beat, his voice reaches a crescendo and I catch myself leaning in, like when I used to listen to the commentary on the car radio.

'And John comes flying out of the backfield to blitz and just flattens the quarterback!'

Blitzing is a tactic used by the defence to disrupt pass attempts by the offence. During a blitz, a higher-than-usual number of defensive players will rush the opposing quarterback, in an attempt to either tackle him, or force him to hurry his pass attempt.

'The ball was turned over to us on that play. As John transitions to offence, they had him go wide out as a receiver and the other team triple-teams him. Possibly in a nod to how fast he was. So, the opposing team knew we were going to throw the ball. And they left the other wide receiver – a senior – open.

Marty is about six foot four and we score, the clock runs out and Hana . . .' He stops, a little overcome with the memory, I think, but his composure is quick.

'Well, you would have thought that his high-school team might have just won the Super Bowl.' The emotion is now barely concealed. 'The stands flooded the field. And of course, my son was a hero.'

John tells me it was such a joy to watch his son play and I don't doubt it, I can hear it in his voice. 'He just wouldn't give up, he had more tenacity than I ever had, and I've got a lot!' he laughs.

He then takes me through John Jr's last game on that field, the soccer match. He played centre midfielder for the majority of the games. This one was no different, only in that it was the quarter-finals that would put the team in the final four of the state soccer championship.

'So, my God, it's cold!' John Sr says, placing us back in the stands once more. 'I'd say probably close to zero Celsius for you, it's freezing, and both teams, I'm not lying, both teams hit the crossbar at least *seven* times each!' He draws out the 'seven' for effect.

It was late in the game, the cold was really setting in on the expectant crowd who were losing faith a little with not a victory in sight for either team, when a friend of John Jr's took a corner kick. John Jr stood on the penalty kick spot and his buddy takes a shot to cross the ball into the corner of the goal, the defender blocks it, sending the ball right back to John's friend who saw John Jr standing all by himself on that penalty spot. He drove the ball about a quarter of a metre off the ground, 'And John flicked it with the back of his heel into the goal and ...' John Sr pauses again. I'm anticipating the whoosh of adrenaline from the crowd to permeate his words, but I quickly recognise his sharp intake as the clipped breath of grief.

'Are you OK, John?'

He clears his throat defiantly, biting back tears, stepping into his role as the commentator in the stadium once more. 'And again,' and his pain is palpable now, 'the place went wild!' He finishes, letting the emotion come. It pours out and I sit very still.

He takes a moment to gather himself and then I can hear him smile. 'There was a big write-up in the paper about him – you know, that was the only goal he ever scored in high school. He was named a Missouri Second Team All-State Soccer Player. Which kind of pissed John Jr off because he loved American football better than soccer!'

We both laugh; we laugh often, in fact, throughout the duration of our conversation. I think of Dawn and Laraine Astle, their humour interwoven with boundless grief; of Karen telling Benjamin Robinson it was a good job he was handsome because his photograph was all over the papers. Flashes of light that seem to spark up and out of the darkness, reminders that life has been lived, that it lived and breathed still. I read somewhere that joy is the justice we give ourselves.

Serving as co-captain on both the soccer and American football teams, John Jr was a leader. He led by example: he wouldn't tell anyone to do anything he wouldn't do himself. He played by the rules. His coaches adored him.

'They would say, if I told him to run through a brick wall, he'd go do it and come back and then ask why. He would never ask why up front. He just trusted the coaches, you know, and he was strong as an ox, swift as a deer, and just had a big, kind heart,' John Sr says. '[He] never started a fight – finished a lot of fights, that's for sure, but never started!' And there's that laugh again.

John Jr stopped playing organised sport by the time he went to college. He told his father he was 'beaten up' from playing through high school. Sometimes he would step onto the pitch at 4.30 p.m. and wouldn't leave until 9 p.m., except to change kits, having played back-to-back games for both of his teams. His athletic talent meant he was well sought after: this was reflected in his positions on the field.

'And those positions are typically getting hit on every play,' John Sr says, 'and you know, later, I found out that there is a study out there that basically said that if you allow your son to play both ways in high school that they can be subjected to up to 2,000 subconcussive hits in one season, but it was long before I knew what I know now.' He sighs.

There were subtle signals from John Jr. He told his father about feeling 'battered', though he never explicitly mentioned his head. 'I'm just thinking, you know, it's his back and his legs and his knees and that kind of stuff,' John Sr says, 'and it wasn't until much later on, you know, I found out that it really, truly was his brain.'

John Jr had had two concussions in his senior year of high school, including one from football and one from soccer, two weeks apart, that were both knockouts.

'So, that's what I suspect was probably the thing that really put John on a downward spiral,' John Sr says. 'But he was a good faker and a good actor, and he kept it to himself until he couldn't keep it from us anymore.'

Concussion had been reared up in the Gaal household before. It was in September 2012 that the youngest Gaal child, Leah, had been in a car with a neighbour and two other children when someone, unbeknown to them, had a heart attack at the wheel and ran a red light. They hit the side of their car, and Leah ended up going to the hospital. At the time, John Jr was just starting his second year of college.

Leah was released from hospital and told to take it easy over the weekend but when she went back into school on the Monday, by 10 a.m. John and Mary had received a phone call saying that she needed to be picked up and that the school suspected she had concussion. 'This is from the school nurse,' John Sr says. 'The doctor in the ER totally missed it. So, we take her back to hospital and they confirm she's got concussion.'

Word of Leah's concussion had reached John Jr at college. He called his mum that night and was very firm. 'I don't care what you have to do,' he had told her, 'drop everything and you see that Leah gets whatever help she can because these concussions from my high-school days have really changed my life.'

John Sr tells me that that phone call had been the first red flag about his injuries but that his son never mentioned them again.

There was something else as well – call it serendipity perhaps, but a little later in the autumn of 2016, the president of John Jr's university announced their September speaker for a yearly event that saw prominent figures from across the globe take to the stage to address students and parents.

'And you're not going to believe this,' John Sr says to me now, 'but it was Dr Bennet Omalu.'

John already knew Omalu from the *Concussion* film and from reading a GQ profile article while on holiday. They had invited John Jr, who hadn't wanted to attend. In hindsight, perhaps he didn't want to hear what he already knew was his own inevitable fate. But John Sr and Mary went along to the talk and even put forward a donation.

'But as I said, this is more from our experience with Leah and not John, you know?' John Sr says.

John Jr had managed to keep his state hidden so it was a shock when he finally admitted to his father in December 2016 that he had struggled all through college, that sometimes he couldn't get out of bed and if it hadn't been for his house-mates, three international students, Mousa, Muzi and Joseph, with whom he had become incredibly close, he's not sure he would have made it out of college at all.

'I hurt so bad every morning that they would dress me and put my backpack on and pushed me out the door, as if I was in kindergarten, like a little toddler,' he told John Sr. When he was in class, he would stare at his textbooks like he was 'looking at a bowl of spaghetti' because that's about how much sense it made when he looked at those words on the page.

'And he said, "My brain's not right,"' John Sr tells me. 'So I said, "Well, let's get you some help."'

The family had tried Western medicine, Eastern medicine, traditional, non-traditional. 'You name it, we tried it,' John Sr says. 'And it was very frustrating for John Jr because every time he went to a new doctor it was a 45-minute interview just rehashing everything he's told five to ten other doctors already and them immediately grabbing the prescription pad and wanting to give him opioids, and he knew that he couldn't go down that path.' On more than one occasion, John Jr called his big sister, Dana, a doctor of pharmacy, to discuss the medicines he was being prescribed.

His symptoms progressed, culminating in 2017 in John Jr putting his fist through a wall in his parents' house after some-thing had triggered him while he was helping his father. It could have been a light going on in the background, a door slamming, music playing, a word that had been said, there was no telling. John Sr had quietly walked away then to pick up his tools, returning to set about fixing the damage. Twenty minutes later, 'I can fix that Dad,' his son said. 'No, I will take care of this' was John Sr's reply. 'We need to help fix you.'

But by then John Jr had fallen deeply. He was at times angry, at others hopeless, sometimes even helpless, his father recalls. It was nothing for him to put his car keys down and then want to go out again 15 minutes later. 'You would just hear outrage,' John Sr says, 'because he couldn't find his car keys. He couldn't remember where he had put them.'

It was a couple of months after the wall incident that Mary Gaal, John Jr's mother, returned her son to the doctor. She was worried and had called the receptionist. The doctor stayed late to see him, putting off a family vacation to Mexico, but expressed his surprise at seeing John Jr so soon since his appointment the day prior. It was now Thursday of the same week, but John Jr swore he was there on Tuesday. Looking confused he said to his mum, 'I lost a day'.

They decided between them that it was time to find a specialist for John. The doctor would see straight to it on his return. Mary had called John Sr who had been on his way home from work. Something wasn't right, she had said; it felt different this time.

'So, I said well, I'm going to call in to work and tell them I'm taking a day off tomorrow to spend a whole day with him,' John Sr had told her. 'We'll do whatever he wants – fishing or if he wants to go for a massage – something relaxing after all this, you know? Get away from it for a bit.'

Shortly after coming home from work, John Jr met his father downstairs. He was quiet when John Sr approached him to ask how he was. 'And I said to him you're not planning to do anything serious, are you?' He didn't even have to say it. John Jr insisted he'd never do anything like that.

Later that evening John Jr announced he was going to the gym to work out. He arrived back home 20 minutes later. A couple of hours passed and he shot up again, deciding to go to his good friend's house to hang out. The family took that as a positive sign, that he wanted to be with an old school friend, somebody he had known and loved for years. He left the family house at around 8.40 p.m. and when he hadn't come home by midnight, Mary and John Sr went to bed. They were awoken around 2 a.m. when their son returned.

'There was some commotion in the bathroom at around 2.30,' John tells me, his voice cracking. He pauses. I tell him it's OK, that we can go as far as he wants to and no further. He swallows and clears his throat, leaving us in silence for a moment longer, and I realise I'm holding my breath.

'At 2.30 I had to bust the door down and he had done some pretty good damage,' he says, expelling the words quickly. 'When I tried to help him . . . he . . . he grabbed my face, you know, still strong as an ox, looked me square in the eyes and just mouthed, "No, Papa, do not try to save me."'

I already know the ending. John Gaal Jr died by suicide at home in Missouri on 24 March 2017, with his father by his side. 'So, I was the first one to hold him when he was born, and I was last to hold him when he died,' John Sr says steadily, a full stop in this unimaginable life sentence.

Unlike Benjamin Robinson, whose injuries were instant, John Gaal Jr's accumulated over time, mostly in the form of concussive and subconcussive blows as a result of tackles or heading the soccer ball. He was strong as an ox, swift as a deer and had a huge heart, as his father had said. His friends and family said his kindness knew no bounds; he was determined both on and off the pitch to help everyone reach their potential. The measure of how much John was loved, not that John Sr wants to put a number on it, was that 1,000 people attended his funeral.

When he died, the family had enquired about donating his organs while they were in the emergency department of the hospital but were told they couldn't be used. 'So, I said, well, I know you can use a couple of them. Do you work with any of the Brain Banks? Do you work with Dr Omalu?' John Sr asked, remembering the talk at the university.

The staff told him that they didn't work with Dr Omalu but they did work with Dr Ann McKee at the VA-BU-CLF Brain Bank in Boston.

'I was like, good enough for me, get me the papers,' he says.

On 6 December 2017, Dr Ann McKee's research team would diagnose John Gaal Jr with Stage I chronic traumatic encephalopathy. I wonder if a CTE diagnosis makes death by suicide more bearable somehow, a final affirmation that there really was nothing you could have done to save your child. What a thought to even have, but it rolls around my head like a marble. I ask John Sr because I have to. He says it did help, but only a fraction.

There was a shred of relief in the room when the diagnosis of Stage I CTE arrived from the lab in Boston. Confirmation that it had been something monstrous that had dragged a kid of John's character to those depths, that he never stood a chance. How deep and dark a hole it had burrowed for him to surmise that the only way out was death. But then there was also despair, that the thing John had loved the most had killed him, followed by the fact that it could have been preventable. He wasn't the first young American footballer player to die by suicide.

A couple of years earlier, 24-year-old Zac Easter, a hard-hitting linebacker from Iowa, had retrieved his 20-gauge shotgun and snuck out of his parents' house. He'd shot himself in the chest, avoiding his brain so it could be preserved and studied. He was convinced he had CTE, having documented his rapid decline in journals and messages to his girlfriend that were later published in *GQ* magazine and subsequently turned into a book, *Love, Zac* (2020). He had hoped that by donating his brain, it might help save someone who still stood a chance, ultimately deciding that his own life was over.[330]

He had left a note for his parents, Brenda and Myles Easter, with instructions to use the money from his memorial to set up a foundation dedicated to studying concussions and to making football a safer sport. His parents agreed to honour his wishes and allow Zac's brain to be examined. It was Dr Bennet Omalu that confirmed his CTE diagnosis.[331]

I think back to the argument by Dr Paul McCrory that there is no evidence to suggest that suicide is a direct result of CTE. I think of BMX legend Dave Mirra placing a gun to his head, of Terry Long drinking antifreeze. While we may not have a black-and-white direct link, there are multiple cases where the symptoms have become so unbearable that ultimately life becomes unliveable for these athletes and that doesn't seem like something that should be left to trial and error or, indeed, further study until we 'know for definite'. I wonder how many more lives it will take before those in power listen?

'The thing that really is so heart breaking,' John Sr says, the wound still raw to recount, 'is that my son died as a result of injuries sustained by two sports he dearly, dearly loved. He would actually be pissed if he saw me trying to dissuade people from playing soccer or American football. But we have to figure out safer ways.'[332]

***

It's often the parents who help, organise, campaign. To say Peter, Benjamin Robinson's dad, has since dedicated his life to raising awareness of brain injury is an understatement. There is no one that fights this cause in the UK like Peter Robinson. After all, a man with nothing to lose is a dangerous one. But Peter chooses his words carefully – online and when we speak – often stating the facts and figures over anything too emotive or personal. But this morning he's made an exception. He posted an image of Benjamin's grave, with the permission of his ex-wife, Karen.[333]

'I'd never posted anything like that before and it did get shared a lot but there was still a troll here and there saying, "He's dead, just get over it," or "Stop making the sport soft,"' Peter tells me. 'I didn't even have to say anything because so many people went for them and they removed their comments in the end.'

The photo was posted an hour before we were due to speak and I sense the weight of that decision still heavy behind his words. Peter apologises for, in his own words, the 'facts-and-stats approach' he has taken to talking about Benjamin, the match and the decade that has followed. He catches my thought before I can say it out loud. 'I guess that must be a kind of coping mechanism, I don't know,' he says quietly. 'It gives me a focus; it's easier to pretend then.' His voice is soft. 'You know, sometimes I'll go out on my bike, and I call it Benjamin time.' He starts, 'If anybody was cycling behind me they would think, *Who is this madman?!* because at times I'm screaming, I'm shouting, just getting it out, getting it out.' He pauses, sighing out whatever he has left. '... I come back and I have that clarity in the head. And then I can go and send another email, do something positive, you know?'

Peter Robinson will go to his grave fighting Benjamin's corner. It feels like the most primal instinct that a parent or loved one can have.

In Dawn Astle's case, the daughter of a man, a once towering figure in their family, who died choking to death in front of their eyes, she fights for him.

'They're not going to win that fight,' journalist Sam Peters had said to me early on in this investigation. 'Sport may not have lost it yet, but they will. [People like Dawn and Peter are] not going away. They've lost the person they loved most in the world. So, it doesn't matter how much spin and bullshit and, you know, denial you throw out, it's like, they're gonna keep fighting and they need their voices heard. And luckily, there are enough people out there who were prepared, and continue to give them their voice.'[334]

'Don't be afraid. They are going to come after you, they are going to call you all types of names – don't worry about it, just speak your truth quietly and clearly and respectfully.'[335]
— Dr Bennet Omalu, neuropathologist

Chapter Ten

The Frontline

I return to speak to Sam Peters in the summer of 2020. He tells me I've found him at a good time. He's chatty because, frankly, he tells me, he's pissed off with rugby. 'Rugby is [a] secret sport in so many ways, like even the art of the breakdown in the scrum and the dark arts that you hear in a lot of what goes on in rugby union. If you compare it to rugby league or you compare it to even American football, it is very hidden.' He adds that rugby has somehow placed itself on some sort of 'higher moral plane to other sports'.[336] Peters suggests this is based around class, and an idea he has heard trotted out by kids all over the world, that rugby is a hooligans' game played by gentlemen, football a gentlemen's game played by hooligans.

'And it's just, it was just a way of, like, emphasising stereo-types around the sort of socio-economic or class backgrounds and different sports . . . [I]t was a way of dividing,' he adds.

Commenting on some of the other factors professional sport has to deal with, he says, 'You've only had to look at some of the incredibly sad stories coming out of British gymnastics in recent times, or the football sex abuse scandal, which the *Guardian* exposed four or five years ago. And cricket's got some significant questions to answer around race and racism . . . I think professional sport in the UK is a tool of control, basically, of organising, ordering and dividing populations . . . [w]hen people think it actually has the opposite effect.'[337]

I ask Sam why he thinks people don't speak out more, why it often takes outsiders – journalists – to dig up stories dealing with these abuses.

'I'd say the worst thing you can be described [as in] rugby union is . . . a "troublemaker",' he responds. 'Within a team or any of the sort of "mavericks" that played, in that they've never succeeded in English professional rugby. They've always been sort of manoeuvred out, partly by the press, who facilitate that role in a lot of ways, but also through a sort of campaign of whispering and, you know, just coaches who won't tolerate any sort of dissent. And so, you end up having this sort of industrialised processing where no one speaks up.'

Sam effectively took one for the team in his 2013 investigation into concussion.[338]

'I don't regret writing one single word,' he says, 'other than, probably – there was one article I wrote which was very critical of how little football had done. And I was probably overly gushing in my praise of rugby in that article, just really as a means of contrasting things. And if I'd known then what I know now, I definitely wouldn't have been as complimentary about rugby.'[339]

He writes on his blog that this process across several years has felt like pushing a heavy cart up a very steep hill, trying to tell rugby's authorities about the obvious and undeniable dangers of allowing an already hugely physical amateur sport to morph so rapidly into a wholly more intense and brutal professional spectacle.

'Am I surprised it got worse? No, not really.'

▲▲▲

Former rugby union player Steve Thompson MBE has requested that we speak over Zoom. He finds it easier to concentrate if he has a visual reference, he says. When we do speak, his wife, Steph, is in the corner of the room, just off screen, in case he forgets anything.

I ask how she has found it – 'it' being the devastating dementia diagnosis Steve received the week before. He's just 42.

'My wife will tell you I've always been a miserable bastard!' Steve laughs, momentarily lightening the mood. It hits me then that by the time this book is released, Steve may not even remember the interview.[340]

Thompson played 195 times for the Northampton Saints before moving to France to play for Brive. He won 73 England caps, and three for the British and Irish Lions, in a nine-year international career. He first retired in 2007 because of a serious neck injury, but was given the all-clear to return, before being forced to retire again in December 2011 with the same problem.

I reached out to Steve, after I had been alerted to a lawsuit brewing against the leading organisations in rugby, World Rugby, the Rugby Football Union in England and Welsh Rugby Union. This was November 2020, a month before it was about to go public. Initiated by eight players, all under 45, including Thompson, his former teammate, 40-year-old Michael Lipman, and the former Wales flanker 41-year-old Alix Popham, all diagnosed with early-onset dementia, it is potentially a landmark case, their claim being that they weren't protected against the risks caused by concussion.

The main objective of the suit is to get families the support they need moving forward, as well as putting together 15 commandments that they would like to see changed. The men are adamant that these changes are for the love of the game. In Popham's case, he had to make 50 contacts a game, each one a potential concussion, coupled with three or four training days a week. The concern from men like Popham and the others joining the suit is that there's absolutely nothing to suggest that the trajectory and the amount of impact that the players go through is going to ease up in any way: in fact, most people on the side of change, whether commentators, players or experts, will tell you it looks likely to implode.

When the litigation went public in December 2020, stories of concussion and brain injury within rugby from current and former players burst out of the press like blood from a severed artery. It grabbed headlines across the country, making waves across the globe. Among the advocates for change are those people who've helped with this book – Chris Nowinski, Alan Pearce, Dr Willie Stewart, Dr Ann McKee, and so many more, all players on the same team.

The suit is a bold move, a necessary one, sure, but it's not the litigation itself that captured my attention, it's something else. For so long the human voice of CTE took the form of the families, the mothers and fathers, wives and daughters, those left to pick up the pieces. Now, alongside them, in stirring chorus for the first time, were the *actual* voices – those with suspected CTE or diagnosed early-onset dementia. And they were young, in their forties, living, breathing, speaking on national television, quoted on the front pages – the players themselves, who know what is happening to them, or what awaits them in the future.

Thompson didn't start playing rugby until quite late, he says, 15 or 16. He has fond memories from back then. It would be a couple of years later that he turned professional and from that point he's not sure if the memories he has are his own or ones he's borrowed from others. He doesn't remember.

One of his most startling admissions that grabbed headlines across the country is that he has no recollection whatsoever of winning the World Cup in Australia in 2003, or anything from the two-month trip, in fact. He's watched recordings of the game since and still can't recall anything. He tells me it's just like he's watching any old England match, that there's nothing connecting him to that game.

'Like it never happened,' he shrugs. 'It's like I've got the camera, but someone's taken the film out. That's how I've got to understand it.'[341]

I ask him how it feels not to be able to remember such a seminal moment in his life, his career. 'I mean, rugby was never my real love,' he says bluntly. 'It was just a job for me. I didn't have any schooling or anything like that, so I got into professional rugby and that's what I've done.'

I'm not sure if his detachment is part of a coping mechanism or just a cruel irony. Perhaps a bit of both. Thompson looks like a rugby player: he fills the screen in front of me, shoulders broad, neck thick and any tell-tale signs that the game has battered him are hidden while he's sitting down.

'I got a lot of problems with my body through rugby,' he says. 'My elbows, knees, sometimes I can't even walk, it's agony. And you go to the doctors, you have tests and they're like, "Well, you're clear."'

Thompson had a lot of hits on the pitch. He tells me he was insecure as a player, even though he was considered one of the best, in the world's top three at one point. He says he constantly felt like he would be dropped or lose his place on the team, or worse, his contract. He felt he had to push harder, play stronger, in order to ensure not just his position but his livelihood.

'Everyone used to laugh at me,' he says. 'Like, "He's just hit his head, he'll wake up in a minute" – and it happened quite often in training, you know: "Oh, just leave him there, he'll, you know, get up in a minute," and then we['d] just carry on, you know, even [in] the matches!'

It's weird, he thinks, that back then, if you pulled a hamstring, you'd get taken off but a whack to the head and it was play on.

'It's gonna be a nightmare when I can't move around properly. Imagine having to pick me up or push me about in a wheelchair!' He laughs again.

I ask him if he has allowed himself to think of the future.

'I am fearful of it,' he says. 'Not for me. I kind of think what will be, will be. I've always been like that. But now I've got responsibilities, I've got to make sure everyone's all right.' Thompson has four children, who have held him to account over his actions prior to his diagnosis.

'My memory was always quite good. But then I'd started to have the odd argument with my wife over something stupid, like I hadn't done something or I thought she'd done something and she hadn't done it, and stuff like that. It was getting all mixed up. And it wasn't until the kids said, "Daddy, you didn't do that," or "You did it." And suddenly you've got someone to back it [all] up.'

It was only when he spoke to Alix Popham that everything suddenly fell into place: 'being angry, the ups and downs', the mood swings – many of their symptoms seemed to align, and Popham persuaded him to see a doctor.

'I always used to be quite a positive person really. And you become so negative. I just felt like this isn't me and it's like an out-of-body experience, really; the downers are horrendous.' His tone is matter of fact as he says this.

Alix Popham had been diagnosed with early-onset dementia and possible CTE, following bouts of rage, including slamming doors until they broke, tearing the bannister off the stairs – actions he had no control over that finally culminated in a breakdown after he got lost out on a bike ride in what he has called 'a total blackout moment'.[342]

Popham had always been told in his career that if he went into a tackle at anything less than 100 per cent, he would be injured. So, he gave it his all three times a week in UK training, then four times a week in France, followed by a game on Saturdays. This would be his routine for 14 years, which his doctor believes means he has accumulated more than 100,000 subconcussions in his career. A hundred thousand.

Alix describes the effects of concussions and subconcussions on his brain as a leaking tap. 'If it drips once or twice there will be no mark on the floor, but if it's dripped for 14 years, there would be a big hole. That is the damage that is showing on the scans.'[343]

Popham is certain that – with the benefit of hindsight – the concussion protocols when he was playing were not adequate.

'You thought concussion was when you were out cold on the pitch,' he says. 'If you felt a bit groggy, you would have a sniff of salts. You didn't want to come off the field as a player and show weakness. You knew your body was going to be sore in retirement, but nobody knew your brain was going to be in bits as well.'

There is a guilt that comes with his diagnosis, Steve tells me: guilt for his family, for his work, but family mainly. 'Am I going to be able to keep working or am I going to be a liability or are people going to be able to help cover for me? And it's like, well, why should they cover for me?'

He tells me he has often thought it would be easier if he wasn't here, though he isn't emotional about it when he says that. It feels like he has accepted his fate. Although, I wonder how much of that is a façade or how much is just his character – another hit taken, ready to walk it off. He is built of strong stuff, that's for sure.

In March 2021, *Guardian* reporter Andy Bull facilitated a conversation between Popham and Dr Bennet Omalu.

Omalu opens the call stating there is no such thing as a safe, violent blow to the human head. 'That is a scientific fact,' he says. 'But because of culture, we develop alternative truths to serve our convenience.'

Popham wants to sit down with the governing bodies and work it out, he says, to protect the game, to protect the players and future generations.

To which Omalu responds: 'Don't be afraid. They are going to come after you, they are going to call you all types of names – don't worry about it, just speak your truth quietly and clearly and respectfully, and let people know you are not against rugby, you just want to improve the quality of life for your fellow human beings.'

It's harder to read when Omalu turns the attention away from sport but to Alix himself.

'I'll tell you the truth, the blunt truth, the radical truth,' Omalu says and I recognise that voice of authority from our conversations, the preacher delivering the sermon. 'We don't have any cure for your disease. All medicine can do for you today is help you to manage your symptoms. What I've noticed, personally, is that retired players who have good family support generally do better.'

Popham responds, 'I have a good family.'[344]

I had watched his wife, Mel, give a devastating interview on the BBC surrounding Alix's own diagnosis.[345]

She appears to be on the verge of tears throughout the interview, the downturn of her mouth a tell-tale sign, yet there is a strength in her vulnerability. She breaks down when she can no longer hold it in, and her cries are guttural.

'It's watching the lights gradually fading in him,' she says on screen. 'My biggest fear is Alix ending up in a nursing home. And for my daughter, my biggest fear is her losing her dad; him being here but not being the same Alix.' Later she reveals that every time she looks at their daughter she bursts into tears. 'How can this be happening?' she pleads.

It's moments like these that stay with me throughout: not the science, not the facts, not the fight, but the people. The people and its impact on them.

At the time of the announcement of the UK suit, the global governing body World Rugby told BBC Sport: 'While not commenting on speculation, World Rugby takes player safety very seriously and implements injury-prevention strategies based on the latest available knowledge, research and evidence.'[346]

The Rugby Football Union, which runs the sport in England, said: 'The RFU has had no legal approach on this matter. The Union takes player safety very seriously and implements injury prevention and injury treatment strategies based on the latest research and evidence. The Union has played an instrumental role in establishing injury surveillance, concussion education and assessment, collaborating on research as well as supporting law changes and law application to ensure proactive management of player welfare.'[347] The Welsh Rugby Union (WRU) said it 'supported and endorsed the World Rugby comment on the subject'.[348]

It feels reminiscent of the AFL's and FA's standard statements following controversy; and yet social commentators have questioned whether this claim will lead to contact in rugby being banned altogether, remarking that this could be 'the end of rugby as we know it' and that the financial implications could be astronomical. This claim has been considered by many to be the key to unlocking a safer future across all sports, in how they tackle brain injury and an interrogation of the actions and education needed to ensure players' protection is paramount.

The British suit against rugby certainly shifted the spotlight from UK football for a moment, though the momentum of both has increased, in part, because of players like Thompson and Popham coming forward.

Following the litigation, on 3 February 2021, World Rugby outlined a detailed return to play protocol that breaks down the steps to be taken should a player be diagnosed with concussion. It features a medically supervised 'six-stage process' that has to be undertaken and states that on completion, a player may only return to play when they have completed a comprehensive neurocognitive test.[349]

An interesting addition to rugby's increasingly urgent player-welfare conversation was announced in the form of a collective of current and former professional players including star names such as James Haskell and current Wales flanker Josh Navidi, sports physicians, match officials and teachers. The group is called Progressive Rugby.

They have stated that rugby has a 'concussion-related existential crisis on its hands', and they want to work collaboratively with the game's authorities to overhaul and improve, in their words, the 'hopelessly inadequate player-welfare safeguards'. The revelation that several retired international players are now suffering from early-onset dementia in their mid-forties was the catalyst for the group's formation. It was launched with a letter to the chairman of World Rugby Sir Bill Beamont, regarding brain trauma in sport, which was signed by 28 signatories with recommendations including an upper-level tackle review, a limit on the number of games a test player can annually play in, an increase in the minimum concussion rest period to three weeks and contact training to be limited.[350]

A statement from World Rugby in response to the Progressive Rugby launch read: 'The welfare of the global rugby family is, and has always been, World Rugby's priority. We take our responsibility very seriously and care deeply about our past, present and future players. That is why we ensure that players are at the heart of our discussions through International Rugby Players, and that is why we value and welcome constructive debate, respect opinions and listen to suggestions that advance welfare.'

World Rugby acknowledged that they too were 'progressive' making reference to Progressive Rugby's name, 'which is why as scientific and medical knowledge and societal understanding continue to evolve, rugby evolves with it. We are always guided by medical and scientific consensus to inform our concussion education, prevention and management strategies.' They said: 'Clearly these members of our rugby family love the game and want it to be the best it can be. We do too. We are encouraged that the group are championing a number of initiatives that are already operational or being considered and we are open to constructive discussions with them regarding their proposals.'[351]

It is true that the prevalence of these social networks also allows people to share research and data more easily. Today, social media has opened up the conversation to fans and spectators in their millions, as opposed to 30, 40 years ago where such discussions would have been limited to a changing-room conversation, say. Now, the global network has opened things up, making it possible for people like Dawn Astle, Peter Robinson, Alan Pearce, Progressive Rugby, along with countless others, to drive the conversation, make the connections, amass the detailed information of those who have been and still are suffering. Those who have been left to fend for themselves, either to protect the dignity of their loved one or because there's been nowhere they could go to for help – financial or otherwise. Often both.

There are certainly mistakes that need to be reconciled with and lessons to be learnt from the past before sport can move forward to ensure a safer and better future. And while it's clear we've already learnt lessons that are too late for Jeff Astle or Benjamin Robinson, this problem is starting to be taken seriously by those that have the power to make a real difference.

My mind always comes back to Dawn Astle, who it seems has been shouting in this room full of people for all of these years, with very few even raising an eyebrow, let alone listening to what she has to say. I wonder if it's been worth it, what sort of impact it has had on her life, flitting between the role of wife and daughter and the head of a foundation. One that lacerates her with grief, the other where she has to keep her head, stay professional.

I suppose we are either defined by the things that break us, or we use them to propel us forward. I think it's both. For Dawn, her father's death has defined an era of protest since, of a fight for justice for something the extent of which we are only really starting to see now, with the countless names across countless sports with countless diagnoses of dementia and probable CTE.

She isn't alone anymore in either challenge.

'Whenever you're asked to reflect on something, it pushes you to consider the journey you've taken to get to this particular point,' Judith Gates tells me. 'I've always been someone who has totally, I would say, believed that the reverberations of the past are always with us. The thoughts and experiences we've had contribute to our motivation today.'[352]

Judith was married young, a pregnant schoolgirl at 16. Her husband, Bill, was a school prefect and captain of the school football team. 'And I think that what emerged for us both was a partnership of equals, which was somewhat unusual in the context of coming from the north-east of England,' she comments. They had two kids; they both worked, Bill as a professional footballer at the age of 17.

'Actually [he was] the first £50-a-week footballer in 1961 because they'd just abolished the maximum wage and he agreed to sign from grammar school as a professional footballer, but made it conditional upon arrangements being made for him to serve as a clerk in order to become a chartered accountant,' Judith says.[353]

'So, he was always highly motivated to have a professional career post-football. And so, all the time he was playing football, he was studying accountancy, learning more about account- ancy. And at the same time, I went to college. I became a teacher. I was rising up the career ladder. I became a head teacher at the age of 29, which was fairly unusual at the time,' Judith says.

They were a career couple and partners. Towards the end of their twenties, two things came side by side, she tells me. One was the 'what next?' in terms of both life and business, which was also prompted by the fact that Bill was suffering from dreadful, dreadful headaches.

'I mean, they continued throughout his thirties to the extent that he even talked with the club doctor at Middlesbrough and said, "You know, have these come from all the heading of the ball?"' Judith says.

This underlying thread connected with heading through- out their life has been a recognition from a fairly early age of the probability and possibility of subsequent problems. Judith and Bill remained in the footballing community and recog- nised that the generation before Bill was suffering. Judith remembers Bill saying to them one day very seriously, 'I could well develop memory problems of the dementia.' The other thing he said to his family throughout those years was: 'If it happens, none of you have to sacrifice your lives for me. You have to make sure I'm well looked after. But you have to keep on living.' That's a testament to his character, Judith affirms, that life was for living.

His decline was slow. At first it would be little things like asking four or five times where or when they were meeting or having lunch. He became less able to deal with complex tasks. They had spent a lifetime renting cars, booking flights, correlating this, coordinating that for their world trips, which he became less and less able to do: 'There was one time in South Africa in 2000 and Bill had gotten into a really confused state about how we could rent a car and where we pick it up from and where we would drive it off.'

'And I remember looking at it . . . and I said, "Just leave it, I'll do it." But I remember thinking, *You could always do that with one hand tied behind your back,*' Judith recalls.

They received his diagnosis in 2014, the same year that Jeff Astle was diagnosed by Dr Willie Stewart with CTE. The neuropsychologist told Bill a sequence of events and then asked him questions. She gave a list of about seven things in a story format.

'I went for a ride on a horse. I can still remember that bit. And they did this and then they saw that. And then she said to him, so what happened at the beginning?' Judith says.

Bill looked at her blankly.

'It was [like] cold water down my back,' Judith says. But then at the end of test, the Gateses were told that they would be very glad to know that Bill didn't have Alzheimer's.[354]

'And it was like a cloud had just lifted, like it sounds clichéd but the sunshine just came through. Then they said they would diagnose him with amnesia, mild cognitive impairment. It can get worse. It may even get better,' Judith says.

She was elated. The Gateses got the train back up to the Northeast all the while thinking that this just might be OK. Until they got off the train, when Bill couldn't remember where he had parked the car. 'And we spent 45 minutes at about 10 o'clock at night looking for the car. It went from the elation of "he's all right" to the absolute roller-coaster of "he's not",' she says.

A couple of years later and things weren't getting better, so they decided to go to the Toronto Memory Clinic. They were in America at the time and the intention was to try to get Bill enrolled in a research project for dementia; they had a whole range of tests, which found that he didn't qualify for the research project because he didn't have sufficient amyloid plaque in the brain for PET scans.

'So even at that time, the head of the clinic and the head of the clinic in London had been pooh-poohing the idea of any connection with football. Then the head of the clinic in Toronto called to say he discovered he had elevated tau. And of course, tau is an indicator. This is something that is indicative of CTE.'

It was at that moment that Judith first felt they had evidence that what was happening to Bill was linked with football.

'And that was when it crystallised, when I talked to our sons, that there was nothing we could do to change things; the only path [was to] endeavour to make his life as happy and as smooth as it could be, but we couldn't change it. And so that was when we said, well, what the heck can we do as a family to try and make a difference?'

Judith did what she knew best as an academic and threw herself into research on sports-related head injuries, on CTE, its history, causes, diagnosis, symptoms, prognosis, outcomes, as well as the stories from families.

'Just how much proof is needed about the harmfulness of some behaviours before remedial action is taken? Just how much proof is needed before dangers to players outweigh maintaining the status quo?' She decided she would come at this from a position of knowledge – as a family member too, but from a position of knowledge. She wanted to gain strength and credibility in order to be able to have influence going forward.

'I mean, I think that there is a tremendous strength in telling players' stories,' she says, 'but I think that there is also the necessity for something beyond that to seek to find the solution.' She tells me: 'The evidence, not the outcomes required by the funding sources, is the ethical basis of research.'

Judith is now one of the founders of Heads for Change, a charity launched by the families of former football and rugby players who have been diagnosed with dementia.[355] It aims to provide support for others with neurodegenerative conditions which they believe were caused by injuries during their careers. As well as empowering independent research into the effects of brain injury, it campaigns to find a unity of purpose between the players, science and governing bodies, which have, until now, been embroiled in battle.

'It's very demanding because I'm always thinking what can be done differently? How can I make a contribution? What knowledge can I come forward with? And so on. But it gives a purpose to what would otherwise just be despair.'

Judith is one of the authors on the October 2021 paper 'Toward Complete, Candid, and Unbiased International Consensus Statements on Concussion in Sport', demanding an overhaul of the Concussion in Sport Group (CISG), which they alleged 'consistently downplay risks'.[356] They stated that over the course of the five international consensus statements on concussion in sports that have been published over the last two decades, their primary finding is that 'the process creating these documents has been narrow, compromised, and flawed. A careful reading of these studies suggests that the authors have adhered to a libertarian framing of causality, risk, and intervention, rather than considering a precautionary, public health and patient-centered point of view.'

They offer several remedies throughout the paper that they claim could help stakeholders resolve the challenge of concussion in sports through the 'bulwark of science'.

One of the points they propose in the paper is for broader inclusion, on the grounds that 'past statements have also included signatories who have consistently downplayed the risks of concussion injury and sought to emphasise all that we do not yet know rather than all that we do know, a pattern that was first established in concussion research for sports by the NFL MTBI Committee which they consider to have ignored the precautionary principle, that scientists and researchers have a social responsibility to act to protect the public from potential harm long before absolute metaphysical certainty has been achieved'.[357]

They claim that the CISG consensus process is both 'biased' and 'unethical' and that it has instead promoted a 'sports-friendly' viewpoint.[358]

For too long 'what we don't know' has given rise to controversy and adversarial points of view. It helps that sport is so ingrained in our culture, the paper notes, because 'as a rule, most people do not like to contemplate their risks'. But it closes in saying that 'no harm can be done by telling readers there are reasons for interpreting and implementing guidelines in a more precautionary way than the centre of gravity of a consensus process unduly weighted by industries with a vested economic interest in the outcome they might prefer'.

It's a bold finish. One that is welcome. At the time of finishing this book, the CISG had yet to respond. I reached out to Paul McCrory personally in regards to claims made within the paper, but heard nothing back.

The Paris conference was supposed to be held in 2020 but was postponed by the pandemic. As was the Paris 2021. It's now set for Amsterdam, in October 2022.

Judith isn't naive about the journey and the subsequent outcome, and is completely saddened at the thought that there will be a time when she cannot protect Bill from the level of confusion and disorientation that he feels right now. She cannot change the reality of her husband's condition. She is, in her own words, losing the battle to retain his consciousness and his very self. I think part of her will be lost with that, the part of her that shares those collective memories, the moments when no one else was around. 'It's devastating in a lot of ways. There's work to be done but there is still enjoyment to be had, still life to be lived,' Judith says.

Judith often walks along the cliff tops in County Durham where they have a home in a little village. 'And there was a moment on that cliff top about two years ago when I went out very early in the morning. I'd left Bill with Nick at home and things were very tough. And I remember standing there and thinking, *I will not let this break me.* But it's now a place of joy because it's a place on the top of the steps that go down over these very rugged cliffs. And we watch the birds together and we have a chat with people who are walking their dogs and engage in a bit of northern humour and all the rest of it.'

Speaking truth to power is a challenging prospect, she says. 'However, even more challenging is the prospect of allowing the powerful and biased status quo to continue. I think people forget that this is about protecting the future, of the sport, but also the players. Our future players, our children,' Judith says. 'That's why we're doing it: for them, the ones that are yet to come.'

The promise of change, a glint of hope on the horizon of tomorrow's grief.

Judith's central tenet, what she wants the future to get from all of her work, is the recognition of the fragility of the brain, in the hope that it will allow us to rethink sport and make minor modifications within it that will protect the brain in the long run.

It's near the end of our conversation when Judith shows me a video of her great grandsons lying side by side on a bed. The oldest boy, Liam, is two and a half at the time and Luca is a couple of weeks old, wriggling next to his brother in a stripey onesie.

'Liam had just learnt a new word from his mum and that word was "delicate",' Judith says.

Liam is looking at his parent behind the camera. 'I can't pick him up because he's delicate,' he says before looking down at his little brother. He reaches out his hand, scanning Luca's body. 'He's got delicate hands,' he says, with a raised finger gently brushing the baby's wrist. His eyes then flash across to the top of Luca's head. 'And a delicate forehead,' his finger hovering just above Luca's skull. 'Delicate baby,' he decides before looking back up to the camera. 'Delicate baby.'

'One can become very emotional, as well as being practical with this,' Judith comments. 'When I looked at them, I thought, all this that we're doing, of course wanting it to be Bill's legacy, as Dawn [Astle] wants it to be her dad's legacy, but I also wanted to protect little boys like those.'

'I've got an image,' Judith adds. 'If you actually think of a wave of change – and that is clearly what is emerging in this situation, a wave of change, a wave of knowledge. We'd actually have to say probably that Dawn was the start of that wave and the wave is gathering momentum and it's getting higher and [there] will come a time when it becomes unstoppable.

'But what happens whenever you have that kind of wave is that you have reaction; you have reaction to the challenge to the status quo. And what you then get is the kind of cross-current, a sort of whirlpool that comes about. And I think the challenge [is] that you have to kind of try and thrive in that cross-current and work out how to get to the whirlpool in order to move the wave in whatever direction.'

She tells me that the power of that wave is matched by the power of the opposition, because almost by definition, it creates an opposition. And it's how you then manage to take something away from the conflicts, when you've got these two powerful waves bashing each other.

'And it actually doesn't get anybody into calmer waters.' She laughs.

I think Judith is right, maybe it shouldn't be a fight, maybe it is in the laying down of those weapons that the greatest and fairest change will be initiated. But it brings into question what roles we are meant to play, what it means to be a witness, and how we each have to question our roles as spectators or indeed the part we are playing in this game.

***

I was a member of chess club at school, out of necessity really, as the single parent I lived with finished work much later than the school bell's last ring. It was something to do other than wait. I was good, not *Queen's Gambit* good, but good enough to hold my own against our teacher, Mr Whalley, who, occasionally, very occasionally, I would beat. Chess is about skill, patience, holding your nerve, always thinking three or four moves ahead, all the while out-manoeuvring your opponent.

The pawns stand on the frontline – ready to lead the play, though always the first taken; the sacrifice you make until the regal pieces who have been sitting proud and protected at the back are ready to go into battle.

The proper moment to resign in chess is when you are losing, or an upcoming checkmate is inevitable. If you are playing against a strong player, it's a good and admirable decision to resign, respectful to their play. It's not so much admitting defeat, as acknowledging there is someone or something better, stronger than you have been. There are winning moves that can be made with pawns; it takes longer and requires more skill but it's not impossible.

I think of the families and researchers who have joined forces and stepped onto the board together, pawns in this game, who are now waiting for sport to make the next move. They've always been waiting.

Judith tells me you can either choose generativity or despair in this situation. She chooses generativity. It's a long game. She and so many others want to protect the generations that are coming through.

'I'm not religious – for me, our mind is who we are,' she says to me, leaning forward and pulling a necklace out from under her collar, 'and when that's gone, what are we left with?'

It strikes me that she says 'we'. And I think about what happens when the person you have built a life with, the persona that is a mirror of you or the person you share a lifetime of memories with, has faded away. Where does that leave you? What is left of you?

'So, I wear this,' she continues, holding out the necklace. It's a question mark on a chain. 'That's my mark, that's kind of who I am.'

Those three little letters, CTE, remain a question mark. At every turn there is new information, new statistics, new insights, new cases and new actions being taken. It exists, that much is true, and yet at the same time the curious nature of the disease means that there is still so much unknown. But for all its mysteries, one thing is clear, that when it comes, there is no turning back. And what I have discovered from the people I have met is that the impact CTE has had, and continues to have, on families is very real.

But what happens next?

It's February 2021 and I'm watching the coverage of the Super Bowl. The Canadian R'n'B singer Abel Tesfaye, better known as The Weeknd, is about to perform the half-time show to an empty stadium following Covid restrictions. After a segment of The Weeknd's most popular songs performed in a funouse-style hall of mirrors, dancers wearing bandages begin to emerge to join him – a nod to the violent imagery in his 'After Hours' music video, which appeared to depict 'the absurd culture of Hollywood celebrity and people manipulating themselves for superficial reasons to please and be validated.'

'It's all a progression and we watch the character's storyline hit heightened levels of danger and absurdity as his tale goes on,' the artist said.[359]

For the finale of his set, the action moves onto the playing field of the stadium where he is accompanied by dozens of dancers, each with bandages wrapped around their heads and faces who line the fields, almost like a marching band reminiscent of American high-school football matches. The Weeknd wouldn't look out of place twirling a baton or cracking a whip like a ring master as he walks down the middle of the pitch in his red, tailored sequin jacket. There's no doubt that despite the absence of a crowd, the stadium is electric; the dancers break out into a riotous final act, throwing themselves about the pitch as the camera pans above.

There is something bitterly ironic, I think, in finishing this book while watching a football field full of people with their heads bandaged. It's a striking final image and it reminds me of Irving Penn's 'football face' image – the beauty and brutality of it I remember Dr Ann McKee telling me, 'CTE has changed me. I don't watch anything in the same way anymore.'

★★★

A phone call between London and the Midlands, spring 2021.

I speak to Dawn for a final time in the early spring of 2021. She's been busy, she always is, and when she answers the phone it's as if no time has passed at all. She greets me like an old friend, launching straight into the conversation as she audibly grapples for her portable charger, her phone already drained of battery from a morning of calls.

'How are you, duck?' she booms, rattling through a cupboard. 'I've just been ringing around because we're doing a Sporting Memories group for some players with dementia, but just players, because normally Sporting Memories is a public thing so we've got some sort of bespoke sessions for players, and I'm just ringing through because obviously some of them aren't brilliant with computers so it's time to do the Zoom and then explain to them how you do it and it's easy enough, they haven't got to put passwords in, they just basically press on the link but it's trying to get them to put the audio on and . . .'

'Not be muted!' I interject, after a year of Zoom calls myself.

'Yeah! And I'm not the best person in the world trying to explain computers! When I joined up with the PFA for these six months and they sent me this bloody computer – I normally work off an iPad which is easy for me – oh my God! When I'm writing out reports it's taking me forever because you have to press the buttons in – I've never used backspace so much in my life! With the iPad if you're not sure of a spelling it comes up, doesn't it? Whereas this, I looked at the word and I don't think I spelled that right, and I'm expecting it to change! Why hasn't it changed itself?! Bloody hell – but I'm getting there. I don't know how in hell I've got this far!' We both laugh.

That Dawn went on to work with the PFA did come as a surprise to a lot of people, but no one was more surprised than Dawn herself.

'It was a shock! I can't even explain how much of a shock it was! I was like, is this a spoof call?!' she exclaims. 'I nearly bloody died when I answered the phone and they said who it was!'

It was shortly after the death of Nobby Stiles that Dawn received a phone call from Chris Hollins, who had been working in communications at the PFA charity for a month. He told her that the PFA recognised that they could have done things better, that he knew they couldn't change the past but that they want to do better. He was ringing to see if she would help them do that alongside her friend Rachel Walden, whose father Rod Taylor, a wing-half for Portsmouth, was also diagnosed by Dr Willie Stewart as having suffered from CTE.

'To be honest, I didn't even have to think about it for very long, I think I rang him back the following day because I knew that it's not about me, it's about the players and the families. As you know, I've been their biggest critic. But when I thought about it, the PFA are a much bigger organisation, much more funded, and they're in this unique position where, I guess, if used, they would certainly have the power to make change quicker than I could!'

The PFA released a statement that announced, 'Dawn Astle and Rachel Walden will be supporting the players' union on an initial six-month advisory basis, to help shape the neurodegenerative care provision for former members and their families.'

PFA Assistant Chief Executive Simon Barker said: 'The PFA has publicly committed to improving the support provisions for families living with dementia and other neurodegenerative diseases. This is a first and essential step, in trying to provide a comprehensive and holistic service.

'Dawn and Rachel's insight and experience will be invaluable to help families both now and in the future. The onus is now on the PFA, to ensure that we fully support them in the next six months and take this opportunity to put in place a long-term care structure and approach.'

The players and the families have remained at the heart of everything Dawn has done; she has taken on a six-month consultancy, though she is clear that she isn't working *for* them, she's working *with* them. The priority is to establish a permanent department within the PFA to try to get them to lobby for a global strategy dealing with dementia and neuro-diseases in football. They had said to her that they would help with funding for respite care, for any home adaptations that might be needed as the disease carries on. They obviously have a financial expert that could help players and families with any benefits they may be entitled to, and they have counsellors if anybody needed counselling, so all these things were in place and it was just made more public and more structured.

Her mum Laraine keeps watching the news half expecting to see the headline 'Dawn Astle walks out of PFA!'

'I said, "No, I'm keeping them on their toes, Mum. I've shouted a couple of times but it's OK,"' Dawn says.

The shouting comes a year and a half since the field study by Dr Willie Stewart, and the PFA have put out another call for a new study to determine why players are three and a half times more likely to develop neurodegenerative disease than the rest of the population. It's almost laughable, I think.

Dawn agrees. 'Well, it's bloody obvious why they are, isn't it?!' she exclaims with a laugh. 'It's not because they play on grass, is it? It's not because of their half-time orange! It's ridiculous!

'If I think they could be doing better, I tell them. I'd spent most of the day doing radio, talking about a causal link, when they go, "No, we haven't got a causal link," something which the FA and the PFA have often preached about. When I speak to Willie Stewart he said we may never actually get a causal link, or at best it may take another 40, 50, 60 years, because the time between what they call the exposure, which is the heading, to the outcome, which is the dementia, can be decades.'

But based on all the evidence that they've got in front of them right now, on the balance of probability, it's heading that's the problem. The field study has answered the question which was set: are our footballers more at risk of neurodegenerative disease than non-footballers in the general population? We know the results. The answer is yes. But now two years on and the PFA have only just put out the next question, which is: 'What's causing it?'

'I mean, why wasn't that done straight away? Why wasn't that question put out as well? And also, if they do this study on what's causing it, they're obviously going to look at heading, aren't they? That's what they're going to be looking at. That's another ten years, and what's going to happen when the results of that come out and they say yes, it's heading that's the problem? What are they going to say then?' Dawn says. 'And we're just going to go on and on and on and on and you cannot do that when people are dying, you cannot do that.'

She firmly believes that football's privileged self-governing status is why it's been allowed to happen for so long, and thinks the government should take responsibility now, or at the very least have an overview of the dementia crisis in football and sport in general. If sport is left to its own devices, the fear is that it will just do what it wants and carry on kicking this particular can down the road for as long as possible.

'We assumed incorrectly that the 2001 research, which obviously the FA and PFA funded, would address the two most obvious issues: how many former footballers have got dementia, one; and two, is the game safe now? And that did neither. It was only our lobbying and dragging the banner everywhere that shamed football into acting.'

Now, however, the higher-profile names coming forward have meant that the crisis is penetrating the mainstream like never before and has brought with it an increased awareness. 'I know people talk about the '66 team and rightly so. Our most iconic team probably forever, but the situation with that team, the fact that five out of the eleven had either sadly died of dementia or are living with dementia, that might sound staggeringly unusual to anybody else but it wasn't for me because I knew there were tragedies of a comparable scale being quietly repeated within all football teams across the length and breadth of the country, who weren't England stars, who played in the lower divisions. I knew there were three, four, five, six players out of the eleven in many other teams. I think, really, the desperately sad news about Nobby and about Sir Bobby Charlton's diagnosis, and especially with it coming so soon after the death of Nobby, I did think it would probably represent a turning point on how it's treated. And it's not right, because it shouldn't make any difference just because they were icons and superstars and legends of the game.'

She agrees that they all matter, regardless of whether they've got an England cap or not.

'I guess it feels more legitimate in a mainstream when it's a name everyone knows,' I offer.

'Yes, and more retired players are commenting about it, who were silent before, which is great, and we were really grateful that the Charlton family spoke out about it publicly because it's not easy to tell people that your husband, dad, grandad, brother is going through this horrible disease. But when families [of] these iconic players do speak out, it does provide extra momentum, it does make people sit up and take notice,' Dawn agrees.

I find Dawn's tenacity astonishing – her drive hasn't faltered even years later; if anything, it's ramped up. Even in the midst of grief, carrying the trauma of not only losing her dad but witnessing his horrific death, she has maintained her sense of humour and managed to keep fighting, somehow finding the strength to join forces with the very industry that took her father away.

'I did it for my dad and the promise I made him, but now I'm doing it for all the other families because it's the right thing to do. I wouldn't be able to live with myself if I'd given up at the first hurdle or not even bothered in the first place and thought what's done is done,' she says. 'It drove me mad anyway, but it would have driven me even madder! It would've been like a maggot niggling away at me all the time, I know it would. But again, I've said this a million times, my dad's death might not have mattered to football, but it mattered to me.'

There are times that she looks back and thinks she should have done more, but I'm not sure what else she could have done when she was fighting against everybody, other than not give up. That was never an option.

'Although, I say that – there were times when I thought, *Jesus Christ, I can't do this anymore*, and I'd have a screaming fit and cry my eyes out and then I'd kick myself up the backside and I'd be all right again.' She laughs 'It's … I don't know. It was incredible pressure and I'll never forgive football for that. I'll never forgive the PFA or the FA for that because this massive responsibility shouldn't have been on my and my family's shoulders.'

★★★

It was announced on 3 March 2021 that MPs would examine links between sport and long-term brain injury in an inquiry carried out by the Digital, Culture, Media and Sport select committee.[360] They would consider scientific evidence for links between head trauma and dementia and how risks could be mitigated with sessions that heard from a number of witnesses, the first taking place on Tuesday, 9 March 2021.

'We will look particularly at what role national governing bodies should be taking, and their responsibilities to understand the risks involved for players and what actions might be taken to mitigate them,' the Committee Chair Julian Knight MP said. 'We're seeing a number of cases involving brain injury in sport likely to reach the doors of our law courts and we will also look at the implications for sport in the longer term of any successful legal claim.'[361]

They heard evidence from former athletes, scientists including Dr Willie Stewart, doctors, players' families, including Dawn Astle, unions and the representatives for governing bodies for various sports, including the PFA's Gordon Taylor.

On Thursday, 27 April 2021, Gordon Taylor appeared before the MPs examining concussion in sport at his own request. He started by outlining football's positive approach to the pandemic, naming Marcus Rashford, but is interrupted by the committee chair since the question posed had been on concussion specifically.[362]

He mentions Jeff Astle then and notes that it was 'something we were very keen to get involved with', citing that they had written to the commission of industrial diseases. He goes on to say, 'Hoping to have some success with that,' though what he means by that is unclear. He states that the research was done but was inconclusive, citing a fall-out between medical experts, though again this was neither interrogated nor verified. 'What we need is a joint approach,' he says; 'it is not just football, it is not just rugby, it is a worldwide issue.'[363]

There is a lot of talk of protecting young athletes from themselves.

The chair notes that this theory is counter to a lot of the evidence they had heard previously from other witnesses who said that 'when they were young, actually, they found themselves pressurized by either coaches and others into not taking care of themselves when they had a concussion. They weren't told to, you know, to leave the pitch, the rink or whatever, but encouraged to get back on and continue'. He says, 'So, you know, which is it?' He asks, 'Is it young athletes being cavalier or is it older coaches and others not having the duty of care that they should perhaps have?'

He directs the question first to Damian Hopley MBE, Chief Executive of the Rugby Players Association, who says that the coach education that's followed and indeed the greater awareness around the area of brain injury now has made a significant difference to the sport. Though there isn't any detail on this.

The responses are often long and digressive, and interrupted regularly by a frozen screen from the intermittent Zoom signal, which causes audible annoyance from the chair, who is already vocally deeply unsatisfied with the answers he is being given.

Later Taylor is asked about claims made by Dr Willie Stewart that football's approach to concussion was a 'shambles',[364] to which Taylor responded, 'I would not agree that it is a shambles, that is a ridiculous thing to say.' In response to the suggestion that his union had been asleep as the wheel, Taylor said: 'We have never been asleep on it. I am perfectly happy to show everyone what we have done, what we are doing and what we intend to do.'

Following the sessions, the committee found that 'unaccountable' governing bodies had failed to address the issue of brain injury in their sports, and said the government had 'failed to take action on player welfare'. The chair of the committee said, 'What is astounding is that when it comes to reducing the risks of brain injury, sport has been allowed to mark its own homework.'

And that the safety of athletes could be easily lost when funding for individual sports depended on how good their protocols looked on paper, but not in practice. It found that there had 'long been a lack of discussion around traumatic brain injuries from sporting bodies'. The report criticises the FA and other sporting bodies in the UK for 'failing to fight hard enough or publicly enough to address the issue of concussion' and concluded that there was 'no overall responsibility' to mandate minimum standards for concussion and head trauma, with each sport left to decide on correct protocols.

They continued that professional sport, like any other business in which employees are at risk of health issues, have statutory responsibilities, but found that these have effectively been delegated to the sporting National Governing Bodies to manage. The report reads: '[F]or too long the sporting landscape has been too fragmented to properly address this issue and government has delayed taking action, deferring to the numerous sporting bodies. We recognise that sport will never be, and can never be, 100-per cent safe. However, the government has a duty to ensure that sporting activity, at every level, bears no unnecessary risk. We recommend that it establishes a UK-wide minimum standard definition for concussion that all sports must use and adapt for their sport.'[365]

It was declared that it was a dereliction of duty, which must change.

'As concerning is grassroots sport with mass participation where we've found negligible effort to track brain injuries and monitor long-term impacts.'

It stated that although science cannot prove a causal link between dementia and sporting activity and demonstrates overall benefits, it is undeniable that a significant minority of people will face long-term neurological issues as a result of their participation in sport and called for a definition of concussion that all sports must use, and a paid medical officer at every major sporting event.

In an official statement the PFA responded to the parliamentary report stating that they welcomed the inquiry and were grateful to the committee for giving them the opportunity to contribute to this report.

'We take the findings of the select committee's inquiry very seriously. Brain injury and increased risk of neurodegenerative diseases in professional footballers is a vital issue relevant to their current and former members and future generations of players.' They said: 'The PFA is responsible for protecting and advocating for the safety and wellbeing of all members and former members. Inquiries such as this – and the independent scrutiny they provide of the footballing authorities – play a vital role in ensuring that we are able to perform this role as effectively as possible.'

They stated their full commitment to using their voice and status within the game to drive progress, awareness and action to support our current and former members. 'The health and wellbeing of our members are paramount, and we will continue working with football's stakeholders to take forward the recommendations within the report ... We are working on a comprehensive strategy to better address the needs of our former members and their families living with a neurodegenerative condition. In the last 12-months, the PFA has started a consultation process with family members of former players and other interested parties to inform the PFA's work in this area, both on and off the field.'[366]

It was reported in July 2021 that from next season, professional players will be limited to ten 'higher-force' headers in training from long passes, corners or free kicks, whereas in the amateur game, players should be limited to ten headers per week.[367]

A joint statement on behalf of the Football Association, Premier League, English Football League, Professional Footballers' Association and League Managers' Association was released.

The preliminary studies identified the varying forces involved in heading a football, which were provided to a cross-football working group to help shape the guidance. Based on those early findings, which showed the majority of headers involve low forces, the initial focus of the guidance [for professional football] will be on headers that involve higher forces. These are typically headers following a long pass (more than 35m) or from crosses, corners and free kicks. It will be recommended that a maximum of 10 higher force headers are carried out in any training week. This recommendation is provided to protect player welfare and will be reviewed regularly as further research is undertaken to understand more regarding the impact of heading in football.

It follows previous restrictions across England, Scotland, Wales and Northern Ireland that have banned heading for the under-12s youth teams.

FA Chief Executive Mark Bullingham stressed their commitment to further medical research to gain an understanding of any risks within football, noting that in the meantime, the rule reduces a potential risk factor.

'It is important to remember that the overwhelming medical evidence [shows] that football and other sports have positive impacts on both mental and physical health,' he added.

A week later, Dr Stewart said, 'There is no basis to say ten headers of a certain level will necessarily make a great difference to the risk. The FA based their recommendations on analysis of matches, estimated what the forces might be and then used that for training guidance. That's like being stood on the edge of the motorway and guessing cars' speeds and talking about road traffic measures in a city. It's not entirely relevant.'

It coincided with the release of his new research, having studied the health records of around 8,000 former players. He examined whether the position footballers play on the pitch and the length of their career impacts their chances of developing dementia. His research found that defenders – who usually head the ball the most – have a five-fold risk of developing neurodegenerative disease and the longer a player's career, the greater the risk of brain-related illness.[368]

Dr Stewart and his team also found that leather and synthetic balls are an almost identical weight and, while the old balls did absorb water and then become heavier, this also meant that they were slower through the air meaning that the argument about the balls themselves is now redundant.

'We are at a point in this current data to suggest that footballs should be sold with a health warning saying, "Repeated heading of a football may lead to an increased risk of dementia,"' Dr Stewart said in the *Telegraph*.[369]

'I would not fall into the comfort zone of thinking modern balls are somehow changing the risks – the risks could actually be higher. Unlike other dementia, and other degenerative diseases, we know what the risk factor is here. It is entirely preventable.'

The responses to Dr Stewart's observation were vast and show just how far we have to go. He's been called a 'do gooder';

others have said there is no need for more 'experts'. Some called it totally ridiculous, claiming that while it was true that when players played with a heavy ball it caused problems, the modern football is very light. Dr Stewart responding by saying: 'Again, the regulation weight of a football has not changed in 150 years.'[370]

It is sometimes hard to reconcile that the thing we love the most might be bad for us. But at what point do we draw the line to say that we have enough evidence for concern?

Football wasn't the only sport to step up in 2021. Following the open letter from Progressive Rugby, in July 2021 the RFU along with Premiership Rugby and the RPA set out the action plan that they have created, aimed at reducing both the exposure-to-head impact and concussion risk within men's and women's elite rugby matches and training in England. The expanded focus on head-impact exposure sits alongside ongoing work to enhance the standard of head-impact and concussion management within the professional game.[371]

In an open letter, Sir Bill Beaumont wrote: 'Like all sports, rugby is not a game that is risk-free. But it is a sport that cares deeply for and prioritises its players, in particular around concussion and head injury [...] In line with our new strategic plan, World Rugby announces the next phase of our player welfare strategy to protect and grow the game we all love. Underpinning this strategy is a personal commitment from myself to never stand still when addressing questions of player welfare. Our ambition is for rugby to be the most progressive sport in the world on player welfare.'[372]

Research conducted as part of the Drake Rugby Biomarker study was released the same month. It was led by Imperial College London and found that participation in elite rugby may be associated with changes in brain structure. The study, which took place between July 2017 and September 2019, assessed 41 male players, and three female players. The rugby players were compared to athletes in non-collision sports, as well as individuals who were not athletes.

Professor David Sharp, senior author from Imperial's Department of Brain Sciences, said: 'Despite relatively high rates of head injury and an increasing focus on prevention, there has been relatively little research investigating the long-term effects of rugby participation. More objective measures of the effects of sporting head injuries on the brain are needed to assist with the assessment and management of individual players.'

Among the group of rugby players, 21 were assessed shortly after sustaining a mild traumatic brain injury, which are the most commonly reported match injury in English professional rugby union, and account for one in five injuries.

The scientists analysed the brain scans for changes in the white matter of the brain and compared these to the athletes in non-collision sports and the non-athletes.

The results revealed that 23 per cent of all the rugby players showed abnormalities to their cell axons (the 'wires' of brain cells), or small tears in blood vessels. These tears cause small leaks in the brain, called microbleeds.

These changes were seen in both players with and without a recent head injury.

In addition, the scans provide evidence for unexpected changes in white-matter volume across the whole group of rugby players, which could indicate a longer-term effect of these abnormalities to connections in the brain. However, further research is needed to understand the significance of these changes in brain structure.

Dr Simon Kemp, Medical Services Director at the Rugby Football Union (RFU), said:

> The RFU is fully committed to advancing our understanding of the short, medium and long-term consequences of head impacts and concussions so that we can ensure that we make continued improvements in player welfare. We welcome any research that helps to advance our knowledge, which is why we actively collaborated with the academic institutions on the Drake Foundation Rugby Biomarker study from its inception, particularly to promote the recruitment of players. While it is unclear from that research what the individual long-term implications are regarding the brain changes seen in these advanced imaging techniques, it is clearly a priority to investigate this further. To further develop our understanding, the RFU, in partnership with Premiership Rugby and independent experts, will be providing a specialist clinical service for the assessment and management of retired elite male and female rugby players between the ages of 30 and 55 to individually assess their brain health. An integrated research programme will review the risk, causes, assessment and management of brain problems for those who have participated in elite rugby.[373]

And yet time remains critical.

In addition to the Biomarker study, the Drake Foundation published a further study in October 2021 that suggested the game may have been safe in the pre-professional era and urged rugby authorities and governing bodies to consider immediate law changes to the sport at all levels.[374] The BRAIN study was funded by the Drake Foundation and published in *Alzheimer's & Dementia: The Journal of the Alzheimer's Association.*

The results from the BRAIN study call into question whether safety standards in the sport have worsened since the game became professional.

They noted that additional research by the Drake Foundation via an online survey of 508 respondents in the UK involved in rugby union had found that 62 per cent of adults involved in grassroots rugby were concerned about long-term effects on brain health, while 61 per cent believe the sport has become more dangerous since turning professional in 1995. Sixty-six per cent believe fundamental law changes are needed to make it safer.

Since the publication of the landmark PFA and FA funded FIELD study, which showed that ex-professional Scottish footballers born between 1900 and 1976 had an approximately 3.5-times increased risk of having dementia as a cause of death, the PFA has been calling for the entire football family to collaborate on a joint response to the issue. They released a statement that said, 'After months of discussions, a draft action is in the process of being agreed, with full details to be confirmed once football families living with dementia have confirmed the proposal meets their needs.' It followed months of talks with the major organisations in the game, including CEOs from the FA, Premier League and EFL, where commitment to this level of support has been provisionally agreed.[375]

At the time of writing this, the final details of the industry-wide care fund are yet to be announced.

In the last two years this story has moved incredibly fast. There were so many seemingly dormant years between the death of Dave Mirra in 2016 and the beginning of 2020, when work and research and diagnosis were happening behind the scenes, the culmination of which is only really starting to gather momentum now and is changing daily in an increasingly public arena.

On Friday, 25 September 2021, at one minute past midnight, I receive an embargoed email from Professor Adam White which details that later in the morning it will be announced to the public that the PFA Chief Executive Maheta Molango and PFA Chair John Mousinho have both pledged to donate their brain as part of the CLF UK concussion initiative backed by the Jeff Astle Foundation.

PFA Chief Executive Molango, a former striker at Brighton & Hove Albion, Lincoln City and Oldham Athletic, stated: 'While being very mindful of taking immediate steps to protect current players, in the long-term ongoing research is vital to enable us to be able to answer more questions and best support members.

'We have been listening and engaging with leading academic experts, and they tell us that brain donation is a key piece to the puzzle in understanding CTE. We are excited to join a global network of the most prominent researchers in this area.'

It came the day after rugby World Cup-winner Steve Thompson became the first athlete to pledge to the Concussion Legacy Project's 'Brain Bank'. He did so 'to make the game safer' so that 'the children of the people I love don't have to go through what I have gone through'.

PFA Chair Mousinho explained: 'Brain donation is an intensely personal decision for former players and their families. However, I have been inspired by the team at the Concussion Legacy Foundation and the Jeff Astle Foundation, and I have decided to commit my brain to future research in the hope that it can help play a part in protecting future generations.'

Speaking on behalf of the Jeff Astle Foundation, Dawn Astle stated: 'Brain donation is the most valuable gift of all for future generations of footballers. It may be many years before this jigsaw is complete but adding each piece, one at a time, is the only way we will understand the true picture and make a better future for others.'

It's a start, but do we wait another 20, 30, 40 years? Or do we acknowledge that the evidence is sufficiently strong enough to consider a sport without unnecessary head impact? There may never be a black-and-white cause and effect for CTE, which feels convenient, and as Dawn said, it could be decades before one is found.

As I write this, reports that New Zealand rugby prop Carl Hayman has been diagnosed with early-onset dementia at the age of 41 start to circulate. Hayman has said he sought medical advice after experiencing memory loss, confusion and suicidal thoughts after retiring in 2007. He earned 45 test caps and played extensively in Europe. The reports state that he has joined the lawsuit brought by Steve Thompson and Alix Popham.

Two weeks later a video was released as part of a new-world rugby initiative, 'The Brain Health Initiative', highlighting the work of 'leading experts' who identified 12 modifiable risks of dementia, only one being a brain injury sustained through playing the game. Other risk factors included depression, a lack of physical activity, lack of social contact, loneliness, heart disease and 'lifestyle' choices such as excessive drinking, smoking or obesity.

At the time of its release, World Rugby, the Rugby Football Union and the Welsh Rugby Union were facing a lawsuit from over 150 former players who are suffering from traumatic brain injury, early-onset dementia and probable CTE.

What they indisputably all have in common is being hit repeatedly in the head over the course of their careers.

Associate Professor Michael Buckland, from the University of Sydney, tweeted that while not the sole cause of dementia, repetitive head injury is the only known risk factor for CTE.

While the initiative is a step forward, this cannot be discounted.

New players come forward each week and I have no doubt that by the time this book is published, the story will have evolved even further. That more voices will have emerged.

That this is just the tip of a very big iceberg.

***

I developed this unusual habit as a teenager of always reading the last page of a book first. Something about needing to know where I was going, perhaps, for resolution, the confirmation that everything was going to be OK. The neat little bow at the end that tied the mysteries of the pages before together, whatever those mysteries might be. But this story is yet to have an ending or any form of resolution. There are questions that still need answering. Why has it taken so long? If warnings were heard, why do they appear to have been ignored?

The biggest question still remains: just how many more players are we willing to sacrifice, and for what?

Since this book went to print, the world-renowned concussion expert Dr Paul McCrory has stood down as chair of the Concussion in Sport Group (CISG) following claims of plagiarism.[376] The Australian Football League published a 260-page report which found that seven of its editorials informed by McCrory contained plagiarised text, and apologised to past players who were 'let down' by the manner in which research into concussion was conducted.[377] In response, McCrory told colleagues that he had made a 'terrible error'.[378] Retracting an article written by him in 2005, the *British Journal of Sports Medicine* cited an 'unlawful and indefensible breach of copyright' by McCrory, who is reported to have apologised.[379] Along with their publisher, the BMJ Group, they released a statement and editorial declaring that their trust in his work was 'broken'.[380]

New research from Oxford Brookes University and twelve other academic institutions, alongside analysis from the Concussion Legacy Foundation, found 'conclusive evidence' that repetitive head impacts cause CTE.[381] However, at the sixth International Consensus Conference on Concussion in Sport, which took place in October 2022 in Amsterdam, Dr Grant Iverson – a neuropsychologist and one of the leaders of the conference (and the beneficiary of $1.5 million in research funding from the NFL)[382] – questioned the work of scientists who have documented CTE in hundreds of athletes, stating that the studies so far did not consider other variables like heart disease, diabetes and substance abuse.[383]

The number of rugby players suffering from traumatic brain injury, early-onset dementia and probable CTE who have joined the litigation against World Rugby, the Rugby Football Union and the Welsh Rugby Union has doubled from 150 to more than 300. That number rises every day. While the fight continues, the cost is lives.

Acknowledgements

It was in August 2020 that I was walking across the cliff tops of Robin Hoods bay in Yorkshire with my Dad during a pretty spectacular crisis of confidence, thinking about how on earth I was ever going to write this book. My mind was in a tangle, I was questioning whether I would be able to bring all the threads and stories together and whether I could do these people justice. I had read earlier that day that Bram Stoker would allegedly stalk the same clifftops, howling into the wind during particularly difficult bouts of writer's block having held an affinity for this Yorkshire coastline given the role it served in birthing Dracula. He wasn't mad, I would realise, he was simply writing a book. Luckily, I didn't have to do it alone.

I don't think there are words big enough to express my gratitude to the people that have been so generous with their time and courageous with the retelling of their stories. Who let me into their lives and living rooms, had countless phone and zoom calls and ultimately trusted me with their words and the legacy of their loved ones. To Dawn and Lorraine Astle, Peter Robinson and Karen, to John Snr. and the Gaal Family, Judith Gates, Steve Thompson and to the women survivors of domestic abuse – this book is for you first and foremost.

To the researchers, scientists, doctors and journalists who have led the way. You are the frontline. Willie Stewart, Michael Grey, John Hardy, Halina Haag, Katherine Snedaker and Pink Concussions, Sam Peters, Eve Valera, Alan Pearce, Lisa Ryan and Ed Daly, Bennett Omalu, Adam White, Chris Nowinski, Robert Cantu, Anne Mckee, Alan Pearce, Alix and Mel Popham, Emma, Kamar, Claire, Rebecca and Craig at G.B.I.R.G. Thank you.

To Harriet Poland, Izzy Everington and the team at Hodder, thank you for your patience and believing that these stories mattered as much as I did. To Abi Bergstrom and Megan Staunton for seeing something in me (like you do with so many others) and encouraging me to write this book. To Adam Strange for having my back and getting me across the finish line. To Tim Crook for the unwavering votes of confidence over the last decade (!). To Thomas Curry, Shola Aleje and Kent De Pinto for your immense support with 'The Beautiful Brain'. This book wouldn't exist without it. To Lauren Eisen for ensuring we got it right every time.

To my family and friends for championing me through the good, the bad and the ugly parts of this process. I love you, thank you, first round is on me. An extended thank you to those of you who stepped into the role of 'sounding board' from the get-go and provided Post-it notes and voice messages, read through chapters and gave me pep talks from various places around the world – Holly, Sophie, Emma, Sienna, Alicia, Bapkins, Leonie, Genuine As, Franck, Fred, Taylor, Biddle, Sarah, thank you.

And to you for picking up this book. For (hopefully) turning the pages and for witnessing these words. The truth only dies when true stories are untold.

Endnotes

Chapter One

1   Ken Liu, *The Man Who Ended History: A Documentary* (Washington DC: Washington Science Fiction Association, 2011).

2   Paul Stuart, 'West Brom: Why Jeff Astle's Daughter Stormed Out of Meeting with PFA Chief Gordon Taylor', *Birmingham Mail*, 20 March 2017, https://www.birminghammail.co.uk/sport/football/football-news/west-brom-jeff-astles-daughter-12767515; PA Media, 'Dementia in Football: Dawn Astle Accuses Authorities of "Shoving Head Injuries Study in a Drawer"', *Sky Sports*, 23 March 2021, https://www.skysports.com/football/news/11095/12254417/dementia-in-football-dawn-astle-accuses-authorities-of-shoving-head-injuries-study-in-a-drawer.

3   Matt Higgins, 'The Last Days of Dave Mirra', *Outside Online*, 17 February 2016, https://www.outsideonline.com/outdoor-adventure/biking/last-days-dave-mirra/.

4   S. Lyng, 'Edgework – A Social Psycological Analysis of Voluntary Risk-Taking', *American Journal of Sociology* (1990).

5   K.A. Mahaffy, 'Edgework: The Sociology of Risk-Taking', *Contemporary Sociology-A Journal of Reviews* (2007).

6   Michael A. Messner, 'When Bodies Are Weapons: Masculinity and Violence in Sport', *International Review for the Sociology of Sport* 25, no. 3 (September 1990): 203–220, https://doi.org/10.1177/101269029002500303.

7   Michael B. Poliakoff, 'Ancient Combat Sports', *Biblical Archaeology Society*, last modified 26 August 2018, https://www.

biblicalarchaeology.org/daily/ancient-cultures/daily-life-and-practice/ancient-combat-sports/.

8   'Boxing', *Brittanica*, last modified 12 November 2021, https://www.britannica.com/sports/boxing.

9   'About Us', *YMCA*, https://ymcaboston.org/about-us/#HISTORY.

10   Pierre Bourdieu, *Distinction: A Social Critique of the Judgement of Taste* (Abingdon, UK: Routledge, 2010) (Original work published 1979), p. 212.

11   Kevin B. Wamsley and David Whitson, 'Celebrating Violent Masculinities: The Boxing Death of Luther McCarty', *Journal of Sport History* 25, no. 3 (1998): 419–431.

12   Joseph Svinth, 'DEATH under the SPOTLIGHT: THE MANUEL VELAZQUEZ COLLECTION, 2011', n.d., https://ejmas.com/jcs/velazquez/Death_Under_the_Spotlight_2011_Final.pdf.

13   Harrison S. Martland, 'Punch Drunk', *Journal of the American Medical Association* 91, no. 15 (October 1928): 1103, https://doi.org/10.1001/jama.1928.02700150029009.

14   Ibid.

15   Eben Pindyck, 'An Obsessive Chronicle of Deaths in the Ring', *The New Yorker*, 22 December 2015, https://www.newyorker.com/sports/sporting-scene/an-obsessive-chronicle-of-deaths-in-the-ring.

16   Martland, 'Punch Drunk'.

17   Ibid.

18   H.L. Parker, 'Traumatic Encephalopathy ('Punch Drunk') of Professional Pugilists', *Journal of Neurology, Neurosurgery & Psychiatry* s1-15, no. 57 (1934): 20–28.

19   J.A. Millspaugh, 'Dementia Pugilistica', *US Naval Med Bull* 35, no. 297 (1937).

20   Michael Osnato and Vincent Giliberti, 'Postconcussion Neurosis-Traumatic Encephalitis: A Conception of Postconcus-

sion Phenomena', *Arch NeurPsych* 18, no. 2 (1927): 181–214, doi:10.1001/archneurpsyc.1927.02210020025002.

21 Karl Murdoch Bowman and Abram Blau, 'Psychotic States Following Head and Brain Injury in Adults and Children', in *Injuries of the Skull, Brain and Spinal Cord: Neuro-Psychiatric, Surgical, and Medico-Legal Aspects*, ed. Samuel Brock (Baltimore: The Williams & Wilkins Co., 1940), 309–360, doi.org/10.1037/11479-013. See also Philip H. Montenigro et al., 'Chronic Traumatic Encephalopathy: Historical Origins and Current Perspective', *Annual Review of Clinical Psychology* 11 (March 2015): 309–330, https://doi.org/10.1146/annurev-clinpsy-032814-112814.

22 Ibid.

23 Charles Bernick and Sarah Banks, 'What Boxing Tells Us about Repetitive Head Trauma and the Brain', *Alzheimer's Research & Therapy* 5, no. 23 (2013), https://doi.org/10.1186/alzrt177.

24 Ibid.

25 Ibid.

26 Montenigro et al., 'Chronic Traumatic Encephalopathy'.

27 J.A. Corsellis, C.J. Bruton and Dorothy Freeman-Browne, 'The Aftermath of Boxing', *Psychological Medicine* 3, no. 3 (1973): 270–303, https://doi.org/10.1017/s0033291700049588.

28 Anthony Herber Roberts, *Brain Damage in Boxers.*

29 Harrison Stanford Martland, 'Intracranial Injuries and Their Sequelae and Punch Drunk', *Ther. Intern. Dis* 3 (1943): 291–301, found in Montenigro et al., 'Chronic Traumatic Encephalopathy'.

30 Montenigro et al., 'Chronic Traumatic Encephalopathy'.

31 Homeopathic Medical Society and State PA, 'Psychoneurosis', *The Hahnemannian Monthly* 68 (1933): 305–306, found in Montenigro et al., 'Chronic Traumatic Encephalopathy'.

32 Health Digest, 'Punch-Drunk Boxers and Football Players', *New York State Journal of Medicine* 36, no. 1654 (1936), found in Montenigro et al., 'Chronic Traumatic Encephalopathy'.

33 Montenigro et al., 'Chronic Traumatic Encephalopathy'.

34   Chris Nowinski, interview with Hana Walker-Brown.

35   Bennet I. Omalu et al., 'Chronic Taumatic Encephalopathy in a National Football League Player', *Neurosurgery* 57,
no. 1 (July 2005): 128–134, https://doi.org/10.1227/01.
neu.0000163407.92769.ed.

36   Ann C. McKee et al., 'Chronic Traumatic Encephalopathy in Athletes: Progressive Tauopathy after Repetitive Head
Injury', *Journal of Neuropathology & Experimental Neurology*
68, no. 7 (July 2009): 709–735, https://doi.org/10.1097/
NEN.0b013e3181a9d503

37   Craig W. Lindsley, 'Chronic Traumatic Encephalopathy (CTE):
A Brief Historical Overview and Recent Focus on NFL Players', *ACS Chemical Neuroscience* 8, no. 8 (August 2017): 1629–
1631, https://doi.org/10.1021/acschemneuro.7b00291.

38   Dr Ann C. McKee, interview with Hana Walker-Brown.

39   James M. Ellison, 'Tau Protein and Alzheimer's Disease: What's
the Connection?', *Bright Focus Foundation,* https://www.
brightfocus.org/alzheimers-disease/article/tau-protein-and-
alzheimers-disease-whats-connection

40   Lindsley, 'Chronic Taumatic Encephalopathy'.

41   Ann C. McKee et al., 'The Spectrum of Disease in Chronic
Taumatic Encephalopathy', *Brain* 136, no. 1 (January 2013):
43–64, https://doi.org/10.1093/brain/aws307.

42   Ibid.

43   Dr Ann C. McKee, interview with Hana Walker-Brown.

44   Digital, Culture, Media and Sport Committee, 'Concussion
in Sport', *UK Parliament, Business, Publications,* 22 July 2021,
https://publications.parliament.uk/pa/cm5802/cmselect/
cmcumeds/46/4602.htm.

45   Bengt Bok, *Encounter with the Other: Some Reflections on Interviewing,* translated by Katherine Stuart, (Stockholm: Stock-
holms dramatiska högskola, 2014).

46   Laraine Astle, interview with Hana Walker-Brown.

47   1968 West Bromwich Albion vs. Everton.

48   Andrew Strong, 'Fantasy Football League – Jeff Astle Sings…
      Hi Ho Silver Lining', YouTube Video, 1:29, 17 May 2010,
      https://www.youtube.com/watch?v=RffriYhX1aE.

49   Steven Morris, 'Heading the Ball Killed Striker', *The Guardian*,
      12 November 2002, https://www.theguardian.com/uk/2002/
      nov/12/football.stevenmorris.

Chapter Two

50   Donald McRae, 'Interview: Dylan Hartley: "Rugby Normalises
      Pain and Injuries – It's the Reality"', *The Guardian*, 28 August
      2020,   https://www.theguardian.com/sport/2020/aug/28/
      dylan-hartley-rugby-normalises-pain-and-injuries-its-the-reality.

51   Andy Bull, 'Death of a schoolboy: why concussion is rugby
      union's dirty secret', *The Guardian*. 13 December 2013,
      https://www.theguardian.com/sport/2013/dec/13/death-of-
      a-schoolboy-ben-robinson-concussion-rugby-union

52   Karen Robinson, interview with Hana Walker-Brown.

53   McRae, 'Dylan Hartley'.

54   Dr Conor O'Brien, 'Bit of a Ruck over the Safety of School
      Rugby', *The Guardian*, 4 March 2016, https://www.theguard-
      ian.com/sport/2016/mar/04/bit-of-a-ruck-over-the-safety-
      of-school-rugby.

55   McRae, 'Dylan Hartley'.

56   Dylan Hartley, *The Hurt* (London:Viking, 2020).

57   Shobhit Jain and Lindsay Iverson, 'Glasgow Coma Scale', *NCBI
      Bookshelf*, last modified 20 June 2021, https://www.ncbi.nlm.
      nih.gov/books/NBK513298/.

Chapter Three

58   George Orwell, *The Complete Works of George Orwell: Facing
      Unpleasant Facts, 1937-1939*, ed. Peter Hobley Davison, Ian
      Angus and Sheila Davison, vol. 11 (Indiana: Secker & War-
      burg, 1998).

59   Peter Robinson, interview with Hana Walker-Brown.

60   Jack Moore, 'Muscular Christianity and American Sports' Undying Love of Violence', *The Guardian*, 8 May 2015, https://www.theguardian.com/sport/blog/2015/may/08/muscular-christianity-and-american-sports-undying-love-of-violence.

61   Aaron Gordon, 'Did Football Cause 20 Deaths in 1905? Re-Investigating a Serial Killer', *Deadspin*, 22 January 2014, https://deadspin.com/did-football-cause-20-deaths-in-1905-re-investigating-1506758181.

62   Bible Gateway, *New International Version* (Biblica, 2011), www.biblegateway.com/versions/New-International-Version-NIV-Bible/.

63   Jan M.I. Klaver, *The Apostle of the Flesh: A Critical Life of Charles Kingsley* (Leiden: Brill, 2006), 371.

64   Thomas Hughes, *Tom Brown at Oxford,* (New York: John W. Lovell Company, 1861).

65   Nick J Watson, Stuart Weir and Stephen Friend, 'The Development of Muscular Christianity in Victorian Britain and beyond', *Journal of Religion & Society* 7 (2015). https://ray.yorksj.ac.uk/id/eprint/840/1/2005-2.pdf_sequence=1.

66   Peter Dixon, *The Olympian* (London: Roundtable Publishing, 1984), 210.

67   Wikipedia Contributors, 'Early History of American Football', *Wikipedia*, Wikimedia Foundation, 15 November 2021, https://en.wikipedia.org/wiki/Early_history_of_American_football.

68   Tony Mason, *Association Football and English Society 1863-1915* (Brighton: Harvester Press, 1981).

69   Mick Cleary, 'Ireland 6 England 12 Six Nations 2013 Match Report,' *The Telegraph*, 10 February 2013, https://www.telegraph.co.uk/sport/rugbyunion/international/sixnations/9852689/Ireland-6-England-12-Six-Nations-2013-match-report.html.

70   David Titterington, 'Muscular Christianity and the Colonizing Power of Modern Sports', Medium, 15 May 2017, https://david-

titterington.medium.com/muscular-christianity-and-the-col-
onizing-power-of-modern-sports-1aa8051b7ec8.

71 'Sport Concussion Assessment Tool,' 5th edition, *British Journal
of Sports Medicine* 51, no. 11 (April 2017): 851–858, https://
bjsm.bmj.com/content/bjsports/early/2017/04/26/bjsports-
2017-097506SCAT5.full.pdf.

72 Sam Peters and Daniel Schofield, 'Rugby's Ticking Time-
bomb! Fear Grows as Evidence Links Brain Damage and
Dementia to Increasing Number of Serious Head Injuries
Suffered by Top Players,' *Daily Mail*, last modified 1 September 2013, https://www.dailymail.co.uk/sport/rugbyunion/
article-2408067/Rugbys-ticking-timebomb-Fears-grow-ev-
idence-links-brain-damage-dementia-increasing-num-
ber-head-injuries-suffered-players.html.

73 Scottish Government, 'Sports Concussion: if in doubt, sit them
out', Scottish Government, January 2014, https://www.jor-
danhill.glasgow.sch.uk/wp-content/uploads/2017/09/scot-
tish_government_concussion_leaflet.pdf

74 Andy Bull, 'Scottish government warns of danger of concussion in school sports', The Guardian, 22 January 2014, https://
www.theguardian.com/sport/2014/jan/22/scottish-govern-
ment-concussion-school-sports

Chapter Four

73 Titterington, 'Muscular Christianity and the Colonizing Power
of Modern Sports'.

74 Montenigro et al., 'Chronic Traumatic Encephalopathy'.

75 Kathryn Henne and Matt Ventresca, 'A Criminal Mind? A
Damged Brain? Narratives of Criminality and Culpability in
the Celebrated Case of Aaron Hernandez', *Crime, Media, Culture: An International Journal* 16, no. 3 (October 2019): 395–
413, https://doi.org/10.1177/1741659019879888.

76 Kalyn Kahler, 'Aaron Hernandez, According to the Journalists Who Covered Him', *Sports Illustrated*, last modified 16

January 2020, https://www.si.com/nfl/2017/04/21/nfl-aar-
on-hernandez-suicide-high-school-bristol-central-col-
lege-florida-new-england-patriots.

77 Jim Gilmore, 'The FRONTLINE Interview: Leigh Steinberg',
29 March 2013, https://www.tpt.org/frontline/video/front-
line-frontline-interview-leigh-steinberg/

78 Mal Florence, 'Remembering the Fearsome Foursome: When
You Think of Defensive Lines, Only Four Names Come to
Mind – Jones, Olsen, Grier and Lundy', *Los Angeles Times*, 16
September 1985, https://www.latimes.com/archives/la-xpm-
1985-09-16-sp-21879-story.html.

79 Kyle Newport, 'Georgia Coach Hurts Own Player after
Slapping Helmet while Celebrating', Bleacher Report,
14 November 2015, https://bleacherreport.com/arti-
cles/2589369-georgia-coach-hurts-own-player-after-slap-
ping-his-helmet-while-celebrating.

80 Mark Fainaru-Wada and Steve Fainaru, *League of Denial: The
NFL, Concussions, and the Battle for Truth*, (New York: Crown
Publishing, 2013).

81 'Stephon Clark: Police Shot Unarmed Man "7 Times in
Back"', *BBC News*, 30 March 2018, https://www.bbc.com/
news/world-us-canada-43598831.

82 Gregory D. Reiber, 'Report of Case Review Sacramento
County Coroner Case 18-01644', *Sacramento County Coroner's
Office*, 20 March 2018, https://www.cityofsacramento.org/-/
media/Corporate/Files/Police/Transparency/Officer-In-
volved-Shootings/Reiber-Review-2018_0422-V2.pdf?la=en.

83 Jose A. Del Real, 'No Charges in Sacramento Police Shooting of Stephon Clark,' *The New York Times Online*, 2
March 2019, https://www.nytimes.com/2019/03/02/us/
stephon-clark-police-shooting-sacramento.html.

84 Omalu et al., 'Chronic Taumatic Encephalopathy in a National
Football League Player'.

85 Fainaru-Wada and Fainaru, *League of Denial*, 448–449.

86   Ibid.

87   Michael Farber, 'The Worst Case: Doctors Warn that Repeated Concussions Can Lead to Permanent Brain Dysfunction', *Sports Illustrated Vault*, last modified 19 December 1994, https://vault. si.com/vault/1994/12/19/the-worst-case-doctors-warn-that-repeated-concussions-can-lead-to-permanent-brain-dysfunction.

88   Don Pierson, 'Heads Up!', *The Chicago Tribune*, 24 December 1999, https://www.chicagotribune.com/news/ct-xpm-1999-12-24-9912240088-story.html.

89   Ibid.

90   James C. McKinley Jr., 'Invisible Injury: A Special Report; A Perplexing Foe Takes An Awful Toll', *The New York Times*, Month Day, 2000, https://www.nytimes.com/2000/05/12/ sports/invisible-injury-a-special-report-a-perplexing-foe-takes-an-awful-toll.html?pagewanted=all&src=pm.

91   Mark R. Lovell et al., 'Grade 1 or "Ding" Concussions in High School Athletes', *The American Journal of Sports Medicine* 32, no. 1 (January 2004): 47–54, https://doi. org/10.1177/0363546503260723.

92   Ira R. Casson, Elliot J. Pellman and David C. Viano, 'Chronic Traumatic Encephalopathy in a National Football League Player', *Neurosurgery* 58, no. 5 (May 2006): E1003, https://doi. org/10.1227/01.NEY.0000217313.15590.C5.

93   Fainaru-Wada and Fainaru, *League of Denial*, 517.

94   JANI v. BERT BELL/PETE ROZELLE NFL PLAYER RETIREMENT PLAN Civil No. WDQ-04-1606 (D. Md. Apr. 26, 2005)

95   Ibid.

96   Ibid.

97   Ibid.

98   Mark Fainaru-Wada and Steve Fainaru, 'Mixed Messages on Brain Injuries', *ESPN*, 15 November 2012, https://www.espn. com/espn/otl/story/_/page/OTL-Mixed-Messages/nfl-dis-

ability-board-concluded-playing-football–caused-brain-inju-
ries–even–officials–issued–denials–years.

99   Bennet Omalu et al., 'Chronic Traumatic Encephalopathy in a National Football League Player: Part II', *Neurosurgery* 59, no. 5 (November 2006): 1086–1093, https://doi.org/10.1227/01. NEU.0000245601.69451.27.

100 Ibid.

101 Jonathan D. Silver, 'Suicide Ruling in Long's Death Hasn't Ended Controversy', *Pittsburgh Post-Gazette*, 26 January 2006, retrieved from https://www.post-gazette.com/sports/steel-ers/2006/01/26/Suicide-ruling-in-Long-s-death-hasn-t-ended-controversy/stories/200601260352.

102 'Former Eagles DB Andre Waters, 44, Commits Suicide,' *ESPN*, 20 November 2006, https://www.espn.com/nfl/news/story?id=2669517.

103 Robert Cantu, 'Chronic Traumatic Encephalopathy in the National Football League', *Neurosurgery* 61, no. 2 (August 2007): 223–225, doi:10.1227/01.NEU.0000255514.73967.90. See also Alan Schwarz, 'Lineman, Dead at 36, Exposes Brain Inju-ries', *The New York Times*, 15 June 2007, https://www.nytimes.com/2007/06/15/sports/football/15brain.html.

104 Christopher Nowinski, *Head Games: Football's Concussion Crisis from the NFL to Youth Leagues* (Massachusetts: Drummond Pub-lishing, 2006).

105 Chris Nowinski, interview with Hana Walker-Brown.

106 Ibid.

107 'Chris Nowinski,' *Concussion Legacy Foundation* (n.d.), https://concussionfoundation.org/about/staff/chris-nowinski.

108 Chris Nowinski, 'Can I Have Your Brain? The Quest for Truth on Concussions and CTE', November 2017, TED video, https://www.ted.com/talks/chris_nowinski_can_i_have_your_brain_the_quest_for_truth_on_concussions_and_cte/transcript?language=en.

109 Michael Kirk, 'League of Denial: The NFL's Concussion Crisis', The Frontline Interviews, *PBS Frontline*, 12 June 2013, https://www.pbs.org/wgbh/pages/frontline/sports/league-of-denial/the-frontline-interview-chris-nowinski/.

110 Schwarz, 'Lineman, Dead at 36'.

111 Ibid.

112 Ibid.

113 'NFL Outlines for Players Steps Taken to Address Concussions', *NFL*, 14 August 2007, https://www.nfl.com/news/nfl-outlines-for-players-steps-taken-to-address-concussions-09000d5d8017cc67.

114 Elliot Pellman and David Viano, 'Concussion in Professional Football: Summary of the Research Conducted by the National Football League's Committee on Mild Traumatic Brain Injury', *Neurosurgical Focus* 21, no. 4 (October 2006): 1–10, https://doi.org/10.3171/foc.2006.21.4.13.

115 Michael Kirk, 'League of Denial: The NFL's Concussion Crisis – Dr Ann McKee', The Frontline Interviews, *PBS Frontline*, 20 May 2013, https://www.pbs.org/wgbh/pages/frontline/sports/league-of-denial/the-frontline-interview-ann-mckee/.

116 Dr Ann C. McKee, interview with Hana Walker-Brown (confirmed via *The Beautiful Brain* ep 2.).

117 Kirk, 'League of Denial: The NFL's Concussion Crisis – Dr Ann McKee'.

118 Boston University, 'Football and Progressive Brain Damage: Tom McHale Of NFL Suffered from Chronic Traumatic Encephalopathy When He Died in 2008,' *Science Daily*, 27 January 2009, www.sciencedaily.com/releases/2009/01/090127165938.htm.

119 Dr Ann C. McKee, interview with Hana Walker-Brown (confirmed via *The Beautiful Brain* ep 2.).

120 Michael Kirk, Jim Gilmore and Mike Wiser, 'League of Denial: The NFL's Concussion Crisis', *PBS*, 2013, https://www.pbs.org/wgbh/frontline/film/league-of-denial/transcript/.

121 Kirk, 'League of Denial: The NFL's Concussion Crisis – Dr Ann McKee'.

122 Kirk, Gilmore and Wiser, 'League of Denial: The NFL's Concussion Crisis.

123 Ibid.

124 Dr Ann C. McKee, interview with Hana Walker-Brown (confirmed via *The Beautiful Brain* ep 2.). See evidence on how sport is worth billions of dollars via NFL revenue 2020): Reuters, 11 March 2021, 'NFL Revenue Dropped by $4 Billion in 2020', retrieved from https://www.reuters.com/lifestyle/sports/report-nfl-revenue-dropped-by-4-billion-2020-2021-03-11/.

125 Dr Ann C. McKee, interview with Hana Walker-Brown (confirmed via *The Beautiful Brain* ep 2. transcript).

126 Jesse Mez et al., 'Clinicopathological Evaluation of Chronic Traumatic Encephalopathy in Players of American Football', *JAMA* 318, no. 4 (2017): 360–370, https://doi.org/10.1001/jama.2017.8334.

127 Rich Barlow, 'Aaron Hernandez's CTE Worst Seen in a Young Person', *The Brink*, 9 November 2017, https://www.bu.edu/articles/2017/aaron-hernandez-cte-worst-seen-in-young-person/.

128 Ibid.

129 'NFL Issues Response to CTE Research Report', *NFL*, 26 July 2017, https://www.nfl.com/news/nfl-issues-response-to-cte-research-report-0ap3000000822159.

130 Mark Fainaru-Wada and Steve Fainaru, 'NFL Takes Control of Brain Research with $100 Million Donation, All but Ending Partnerships with Outside Entities', *ESPN*, 31 August 2017, https://www.espn.co.uk/espn/otl/story/_/id/20509977/nfl-takes-control-brain-research-100-million-donation-all-ending-partnerships-entities.

131 Dr Ann C. McKee, interview with Hana Walker-Brown.

132 Chris Nowinski, interview with Hana Walker-Brown.

Chapter Five

133 Bram Endedijk and Enzo van Steenbergen, 'Evidence of Brain Damage, but Sports Associations Look Away', NRC, 23 October 2020, https://www.nrc.nl/nieuws/2020/10/23/deny-ignore-frustrate-a4017146.

134 *Gladiator*, directed by Ridley Scott (DreamWorks Distribution, 2000).

135 Alan J. Pearce et al., 'Chronic Traumatic Encephalopathy in a Former Australian Rules Football Player Diagnosed with Alzheimer's Disease', *Acta Neuropathologica Communications* 8, no. 1 (2020): 23, doi:10.1186/s40478-020-0895-z.

136 Stated in interview with Alan J. Pearce – 14:27, 4 November 2020 and confirmed via 1997 official media statement from transport minister: 'Transport Minister Eric Charlton today announced that the city's northern bypass would be officially named the Graham Farmer Freeway in honour of one of the State's greatest and best-known sporting identities.' 'N. Bypass to Be Officially Renamed the Grham Farmer Freeway', Media Statements, *Government of Western Australia*, 6 October 1997, https://www.mediastatements.wa.gov.au/Pages/Court/1997/10/NBypass-to-be-officially-named-the-Graham-Farmer-Freeway.aspx. See also 'Northbridge Tunnel', *Mainroads West Australia*, https://www.mainroads.wa.gov.au/travel-information/driving-in-wa/driving-in-perth/northbridge-tunnel/.

137 'Alzheimer's Disease Facts and Figures', *Alzheimer's & Dementia* 15, no. 3 (2019), doi:10.1016/j.jalz.2019.01.010.

138 Pearce et al., 'Chronic Traumatic Encephalopathy'.

139 Amanda Rush and Greg Sutherland, 'The Future of Brain Banking in Australia: An Integrated Brain and Body Biolibrary,' *Medical Journal of Australia* 214, no. 10 (June 2021): 447–449, doi:10.5694/mja2.51049.

140 Jourdan Canill, '"We'll Continue to Learn": AFL on "Polly" Farmer's CTE Diagnosis', *AFL*, 27 February 2020, https://

www.afl.com.au/news/378562/well-continue-to-learn-afl-on-polly-farmers-cte-diagnosis.

141 Canill, 'We'll Continue to Learn'.

142 Cindy Boren, 'Aaron Hernandez's Murder Conviction Reinstated by Massachusetts's Highest Court', *The Washington Post*, 13 March 2019, https://www.washingtonpost.com/sports/2019/03/13/aaron-hernandezs-murder-conviction-reinstated-by-massachusettss-highest-court/.

143 Aja Romano, 'Netflix's Flawed Aaron Hernandez Documentary Raises More Questions Than It Answers', *Vox*, 2 February 2020, https://www.vox.com/culture/2020/2/2/21116353/aaron-hernandez-life-netflix-documentary-killer-inside-review.

144 'Danny Frawley Was Suffering from Concussion-Linked Brain Condition at Time of Death, AFL Thanks Family for Allowing Research - ABC News', *ABC News*, 31 August 2020, https://www.abc.net.au/news/2020-09-01/danny-frawley-was-suffering-from-cte-at-time-of-death/12615774.

145 Sam Goodwin, 'Coroner Confirms Devastating Details in Danny Frawley's Tragic Death', *Yahoo Sport*, 23 February 2021, https://au.sports.yahoo.com/afl-2021-coroner-confirms-sad-details-danny-frawley-death-194515191.html?guccounter=1. See also 'Coroner's Report Reveals Sad Details of Late AFL Great Frawley's Death', *Fox Sports*, 23 February 2021, https://www.foxsports.com.au/afl/afl-2021-danny-frawley-coroners-report-death-depression-mental-health-battle-details-latest-news/news-story/ed3d84adf09d2da6dc-9c74bc99f17562.

146 Paresa Antoniadis Spanos, 'Finding into Death without Inquest COR 2019 4895', Coroner's Court of Victoria, Melbourne, https://www.coronerscourt.vic.gov.au/sites/default/files/2021-02/Finding D Frawley.pdf

147 https://www.heraldsun.com.au/sport/afl/danny-frawley-suffered-from-brain-disorder-chronic-traumatic-encephalop-

athy-known-as-cte/news-story/fbd5b5fd989a2bd51fced-cd36197b177.

148 Michael E. Buckland et al., 'Chronic Traumatic Encephalopa-thy in Two Former Australian National Rugby League Players,' *Acta Neuropathologica Communications* 7, no. 1 (June 2019): 97, doi:10.1186/s40478-019-0751-1.

149 Adam Pengilly, '"Significant Share" of Ex-Players Likely to Have CTE, Warns Concussion Expert,' *The Sunday Morning Herald*, 27 June 2019, https://www.smh.com.au/sport/nrl/significant-share-of-ex-players-likely-to-have-cte-warns-con-cussion-expert-20190627-p521vy.html.

150 Margie McDonald, 'Brainstorm: Eels Greats Set to Follow Sterlo's Lead,' *NRL*, 28 June 2019, https://www.nrl.com/news/2019/06/28/brainstorm-eels-greats-set-to-follow-ster-los-lead/.

151 McDonald, 'Brainstorm'.

152 Alan Pearce, interview with Hana Walker-Brown, November 2020, 10:07.

153 'AFL Statement on Updated Concussion Guidelines', *AFLW*, 2021, https://www.womens.afl/news/56964/afl-statement-on-updated-concussion-guidelines. See also Callum Twomey, 'AFL Doubles Mandatory Break under Strict New Concussion Protocols', *AFL*, 28 January 2021, https://www.afl.com.au/news/543220/afl-doubles-mandatory-break-under-strict-new-concussion-protocols.

154 Michael Warner, 'Neuroscientist Reveals Alarming Results from Concussion Study on Retired VFL/AFL Players', *The Australian*, 12 April 2021, https://www.theaustralian.com.au/sport/afl/news/neuroscientist-reveals-alarming-re-sults-from-concussion-study-on-retired-vflafl-players/news-story/e51ffe9937bb1f48af648241d740d020.

155 Alan Pearce, interview with Hana Walker-Brown, 4 November 2020.

156 Ibid.

157 Louise Milligan, 'These Are the Sporting Clashes Having a Disastrous Impact', *ABC Australia*, 8 October 2015, https://www.abc.net.au/7.30/these-are-the-sporting-clashes-having-a-disastrous/6843244.

158 Tim Dodd and Paul McCarthy, 'The Austrlian's Research Magazine Takes a Deep Dive into Research', *The Weekend Australian*, 10 November 2021, https://www.theaustralian.com.au/special-reports/the-australians-...p-dive-into-research/news-story/6bde9f53e5846a150a25abe7758adedd.

159 The Florey Institute of Neuroscience and Mental Health, 'The Concussion "Crisis" – Media, Myths and Medicine' by Paul McCrory, YouTube Video, 7 April 2016, https://www.youtube.com/watch?v=oPrpTj2Edp8.

160 patrickw@themonthly.com.au, 'The AFL's Concussion Problem | Wendy Carlisle', *The Monthly*, 31 August 2018, https://www.themonthly.com.au/issue/2018/september/1535724000/wendy-carlisle/afl-s-concussion-problem#mtr.

161 The Florey Institute, 'The Concussion "Crisis"'.

162 *The Florey Annual 2015–2016*, p. 5, Florey Institute of Neuroscience and Mental Health.

163 'Definition of "Myth"', *Merriam-Webster*, last modified 19 November 2021, https://www.merriam-webster.com/dictionary/myth.

164 Paul McCrory, 'The Eighth Wonder of the World: The Mythology of Concussion Management', *British Journal of Sports Medicine* 33, no. 2 (April 1999): 136–137, doi:10.1136/bjsm.33.2.136.

165 Gavin A. Davis, Rudolph J. Castellani and Paul McCrory, 'Neurodegeneration and Sport,' *Neurosurgery* 76, no. 6 (June 2015): 643–656, doi:10.1227/NEU.0000000000000722.

166 Paul McCrory et al., 'Does "Second Impact Syndrome" Exist?', in *The Oxford Handbook of Sports-Related Concussion*, ed. Ruben Echemendia and Grant L. Iverson (Oxford: Oxford University Press, 2015), doi:10.1093/oxfordhb/9780199896585.013.001.

167   Ibid.

168   Charles Tator et al., 'Fatal Second Impact Syndrome in Rowan Stringer, A 17-Year-Old Rugby Player', *The Canadian Journal of Neurological Sciences. Le journal canadien des sciences neurologiques* 46, no. 3 (May 2019): 351–354, https://doi.org/10.1017/cjn.2019.14.

169   'International Symposium on Concussion in Sport', *BJ Sport Med* (2001): 367-377, https://bjsm.bmj.com/content/bjsports/35/5/367.full.pdf.

170   Mark Aubry et al., 'Summary and Agreement Statement of the First International conference on Concussion in Sport, Vienna 2001', *The Physician and Sportsmedicine* 30, no. 2 (2002): 57–63, doi:10.3810/psm.2002.02.176.

171   Margaret Pusateri, Brandon Hockenberry and Chirstopher McGrew, 'Zurich to Berlin "Where" Are We Now with the Concussion in Sport Group?', *Current Sports Medicine Reports* 17, no. 1 (January 2018): 26–30, https://doi.org/10.1249/JSR.0000000000000444.

172   Paul McCrory et al., 'Consensus Statement on Concussion in Sport - the 5th International Conference on Concussion in Sport Held in Berlin, October 2016', *British Journal of Sports Medicine* 51, no. 11 (May 2017): 838–847, https://doi.org/10.1136/bjsports-2017-097699.

173   'The Management of Concussion', Operations, *NRL*, https://www.nrl.com/operations/the-players/management-of-concussion/.

174   Bram Endedijk and Enzo van Steenbergen, 'Evidence of Brain Damage, but Sports Associations Look Away', NRC, 23 October 2020, https://www.nrc.nl/nieuws/2020/10/23/deny-ignore-frustrate-a4017146. See also Andy Bull, 'Families of Jack Charlton and Nobby Stiles Back New Concussion Campaign,' Sport, *The Guardian*, 24 October 2020, https://www.theguardian.com/sport/2020/oct/24/families-of-jack-charlton-and-nobby-stiles-back-new-concussion-dementia-cam-

paign. See also Jeremy Allingham, 'Brain Trust: Big Questions Surround the Most Influential Concussion Research on the Planet', *CBC News*, 2 March 2020, https://newsinteractives. cbc.ca/longform/brain-trust.

175   Jeremy Allingham, 'Brain Trust: How B.C.'s Sports Organizations Are Facing the Concussion Epidemic', *CBC News*, 5 March 2020, https://www.cbc.ca/news/canada/british-columbia/brain-trust-grassroots-1.5485443.

176   Ibid.

177   Alan Pearce, interview with Hana Walker-Brown, 40:33.

178   Alan Pearce, interview with Hana Walker-Brown, 45:33.

179   Ibid.

Chapter Six

180   'Brisbane Lions Defender Justin Clarke Quits AFL at 22, After Training Accident Leaves Him with Serious Concussion and Memory Issues', *ABC Australia*, 31 March 2016, https://www. abc.net.au/news/2016-03-31/lions-justin-clarke-retires-at-22-over-serious-concussion/7288464.

181   Adrian Proszenko, 'World-First Study of League Players Finds No Link between Concussions and Depression Risk', *The Sunday Morning Herald*, 24 October 2021, https://www.smh.com.au/sport/nrl/world-first-study-of-league-players-finds-no-link-between-concussions-and-depression-risk-20211023-p592ic.html.

182   Kat Czekaj, interview with Hana Walker-Brown.

183   Ibid.

184   Proscenko, 'World-First Study of League Players'.

185   See Chapter Three, page 62

186   Sam Peters, interview with Hana Walker-Brown.

187   Ibid.

188   Ibid.

189   Sam Peters and Daniel Schofield, 'Rugby's Ticking Time-bomb! Fears Grow as Evidence Links Brain Damage and Dementia to Increasing Number of Serious Head Injuries Suf-

fered by Top Players', Mail on Sunday, *Daily Mail*, 31 August 2013, https://www.dailymail.co.uk/sport/rugbyunion/article-2408067/Rugbys-ticking-timebomb-Fears-grow-evidence-links-brain-damage-dementia-increasing-number-head-injuries-suffered-players.html.

190 Peters and Schofield, 'Rugby's Ticking Timebomb!'

191 Robin Scott-Elliot, 'The Big Question: Why Has Rugby Union Become So Dangerous, and What Should Be Done?', *The Independent*, 4 November 2009, https://www.independent.co.uk/sport/rugby/rugby-union/news-comment/the-big-question-why-has-rugby-union-become-so-dangerous-and-what-should-be-done-1814152.html.

192 'The Drake Foundation Urges Immediate Changes in Rugby to Further Prioritise Player Welfare', latest News, *The Drake Foundation*, 22 July 2021, https://www.drakefoundation.org/the-drake-foundation-urges-immediate-changes-in-rugby-to-further-prioritise-player-welfare/.

193 Sam Peters, interview with Hana Walker-Brown.

194 Johnny Watterson, 'Concussion Issue Big Enough but Now Research Links Big Hits with Alzheimer's', *The Irish Times*, 31 August 2013, https://www.irishtimes.com/sport/concussion-issue-big-enough-but-now-research-links-big-hits-with-alzheimer-s-1.1511018.

195 'Study Reveals Dementia Risk in Former Professional Footballers', University News, University of Glasgow, 21 October 2019, https://www.gla.ac.uk/news/archiveofnews/2019/october/headline_681082_en.html.

196 Dr Willie Stewart, interview with Hana Walker-Brown.

197 Ibid.

198 Ibid.

199 https://www.reuters.com/article/us-usa-crime-hernandez-idUSKCN1BW2LN. See also official document: http://i2.cdn.turner.com/cnn/2017/images/09/21/hernandez.v..national.football.league.et.al.-.pacer.1.complaint.pdf.

200 https://www.reuters.com/article/us-usa-crime-hernan-dez-idUSKCN1BX2NP.

201 https://cdn1.sportngin.com/attachments/docu-ment/0054/0269/RIDDELL__06_19_13.pdf.

202 https://uspto.report/patent/app/20190254378.

203 Brett Zaroa, 'Gridiron Gear Goes to War', *Popular Science* 273, no. 3 (2008): 86.

204 https://casetext.com/case/in-re-riddell-concussion-reduc-tion-litig-5#N196815.

205 https://drive.google.com/file/d/1MooMepavgloKxJmNVz-ri41aJ79EGzetU/view.

206 https://apnews.com/article/0fb9756a42e0472eadb05b339d-1bcb15.

207 The 42, 'If you're worried about the physical side of any sport, then play chess', 3 October 2017, https://www.the42.ie/roy-keane-physical-side-sport-chess-3627845-Oct2017/

208 Michael Perelman and Vincent Portillo, *The Matrix: An Explora-tion of the Interactions between the Economy, War, and Economic Theory.*

209 Hartley, *The Hurt.*

210 Marc Edwards, *RugbyPass Offload*, Apple Podcast, https://pod-casts.apple.com/gb/podcast/rugbypass-offload/id1533365390.

211 Fivealex2010, 'The Agony of Defeat, Jim McKay', You-Tube video, 23 February 2010, https://www.youtube.com/watch?v=i1mFGrqytaI.

Chapter Seven

212 Illya McLellan, 'The Cult of Football: A Religion for the Twentieth Century and Beyond', *Bleacher Report*, 20 September 2008, https://bleacherreport.com/articles/59738-the-cultof-football-a-religion-for-the-twentieth-century-and-beyond.

213 Asif Kapadia, *Diego Maradona*, directed by Asif Kapadia (UK: On the Corner Film4, 2019).

214 Ibid.

215 Professional Footballers' Association, 'Call for Evidence: Concussion in Sport Written Evidence,' *UK Parliament* (N.D.), https://committees.parliament.uk/writtenevidence/25350/html/.

216 Laraine Astle, interview with Hana Walker-Brown.

217 Dawn Astle, interview with Hana Walker-Brown.

218 Ibid.

219 Sam Peters, 'Exclusive: Jeff Astle's Family Accuse Football's Authorities after Ex-England Striker Died from Same Disease Found in Brain-Damaged Boxers', *Daily Mail Online*, last modified 2 June 2014, https://www.dailymail.co.uk/sport/concussion/article-2644983/EXCLUSIVE-Jeff-Astles-family-accuse-authorities-ex-England-striker-died-disease-kills-brain-damaged-boxers-American-footballers.html.

220 Sam Peters, interview with Hana Walker-Brown.

221 Sam Peters, 'Football in the Dock amid Confusion over FA's Promise of a 10-Year Study on Link between Football and Dementia', *Daily Mail Online*, last modified 4 April 2014, https://www.dailymail.co.uk/sport/football/article-2586987/Football-dock-amid-confusion-FAs-promise-10-year-study-link-football-dementia.html.

222 Ibid.

223 See footage of Burnley tribute: DavoBirmingham2, 'Blues & West Brom Fans Pay Tribute to Jeff Astle', YouTube video, 25 January 2015, https://www.youtube.com/watch?v=o-j6kvwxJ57k.

224 Dawn Astle, interview with Hana Walker-Brown.

225 Ibid.

226 Mike Keegan, 'Revealed: Doc's Dementia Warning was Ignored... 24 Years Ago', *Pressreader*, 3 December 2020, https://www.pressreader.com/uk/daily-mail/20201203/283875870733848.

227 'Doctor who first raised dementia alarm 24 Years Ago was fobbed off by the FA and Premier League,' *Express Digest,* (n.d.), https://expressdigest.com/doctor-who-first-raised-de-

mentia-alarm-24-years-ago-was-fobbed-off-by-the-fa-and-premier-league/

228 Letter from Mike Sadler.

229 Statement emailed to author.

230 Jeremy Wilson, 'PFA "ignored" doctor's warning over brain damage in 1993', The Daily Telegraph, 21 March 2018, https://www.telegraph.co.uk/football/2018/03/20/pfa-ignored-doctors-warning-brain-damage-1993/

231 Kieran Gill, 'Exclusive: FIFA's Dementia Shame: Governing Body Knew about Football's Brain Damage Link in 1984 When Their Own Magazine Highlighted Heading Dangers... So, Why Did They Ignore the Warnings?', The Daily Mail Online, last modified 6 October 2021, https://www.dailymail.co.uk/sport/sports-news/article-10062039/FIFAs-dementia-SHAME-Governing-body-knew-footballs-brain-damage-link-1984.html.

232 'Employment Tribunal Explained', 2013, Explained.today, https://everything.explained.today/Employment_tribunal/.

233 'BBC News | SCOTLAND | Transcript: Heading for Trouble', 2021, BBC, http://news.bbc.co.uk/1/hi/scotland/732497.stm.

234 Ibid.

235 Ibid.

236 Sam Peters, 'FA Chairman Greg Dyke Apologises to Jeff Astle's Family and Pledges to Fund Research into Head Injuries', Mail on Sunday, The Daily Mail Online, last modified 12 April 2015, https://www.dailymail.co.uk/sport/football/article-3035360/FA-chairman-Greg-Dyke-apologises-Jeff-Astle-s-family-pledges-fund-research-head-injuries.html.

237 Ibid.

238 Laraine Astle, interview with Hana Walker-Brown.

239 'NFL, Retired Players Resolve Concussion Litigation; Court-Appointed Mediator Hails "Historic" Agreement' (Newport: Alternative Dispute Resolution Cen-

tre), n.d., http://static.nfl.com/static/content/public/pho-to/2013/08/29/0ap2000000235504.pdf.

240 Ibid.

241 'NFL, Ex-Players Agree to $765M Settlement in Concussions Suit', *NFL*, 29 August 2013, https://www.nfl.com/news/nfl-ex-players-agree-to-765m-settlement-in-concussions-suit-0ap1000000235494.

242 'Timeline: The NFL's Concussion Crisis – League of Denial: The NFL's Concussion Crisis - FRONTLINE', *FRONT-LINE*, 2013, https://www.pbs.org/wgbh/pages/frontline/sports/league-of-denial/timeline-the-nfls-concussion-cri-sis/.

243 'Injury Data since 2015', *NFL*, 2015, https://www.nfl.com/playerhealthandsafety/health-and-wellness/injury-data/injury-data.

244 Chris Nowinski, interview with Hana Walker-Brown.

245 'FA and PFA Commission New Study into Risk of Demen-tia from Playing Football', *The Independent*, 23 November 2017, https://www.independent.co.uk/sport/football/pre-mier-league/dementia-in-football-fa-pfa-report-investiga-tion-study-heading-a8071426.html.

246 Ibid.

247 'Study Reveals Dementia Risk in Former Professional Foot-ballers', *University News*, University of Glasgow.

Chapter Eight

248 *Roll Red Roll,* directed by Nancy Schwartzman (Chicago: Together Films, 2018).

249 Ella, interview with Hana Walker-Brown.

250 *Vogue* Magazine, 'Put On Your Game Face. Photographed by Irving Penn, styled by @phyllis_posnick', Instagram, 5 Febru-ary 2017, https://www.instagram.com/p/BQJgCzfguPz/?tak-en-by=voguemagazine.

251   *Vogue* Magazine, 'Superbowl Sunday Is Officially Here', Instagram, 7 February 2021, https://www.instagram.com/p/CLAIAQdlapL/.

252   Irving Penn Centennial; Metropolitan Museum of Arts, New York; notes from the exhibition.

253   Ibid.

254   Neil K. McGroarty, Symone M. Brown and Mary K. Mulcahey, 'Sport-Related Concussion in Female Athletes: A Systematic Review', *Orthopaedic Journal of Sports Medicine* 8, no. 7 (July 2020), https://doi.org/10.1177/2325967120932306.

255   'Male and Female Brains Respond to Injury Differently, Research Shows', *The Independent*, 17 December 2019, https://www.independent.co.uk/news/long_reads/male-female-brains-injury-different-research-study-a9233086.html?r=91568.

256   'Study Links Menstrual Cycle, Concussion Outcomes in Women', News, *University of Rochester Medical Center*, 13 November 2003, https://www.urmc.rochester.edu/news/story/study-links-menstrual-cycle-concussion-outcomes-in.

257   Blessen C. Eapen et al., 'Rehabilitation of Moderate-to-Severe Traumatic Brain Injury', *Semin Neurol* 35, no. 1 (February 2015): 1–13, doi:10.1055/s-0035-1549094.

258   George Washington Roberts et al., 'Dementia in a Punch-Drunk Wife', *The Lancet* 335 (1990): 918–919, doi: 10.1016/0140-6736(90)90520-f.

259   Ibid.

260   Jennifer Crane, 'The Battered Child Syndrome: Parents and Children as Objects of Medical Study', in *Child Protection in England, 1960–2000: Expertise, Experience, and Emotion* (London: Palgrave Macmillan, 2018).

261   Steven J. Kirsh, 'Cartoon Violence and Aggression in Youth', *Aggression and Violent Behavior* 11, no. 6 (2006): 547–557, https://doi.org/10.1016/j.avb.2005.10.002.

262   James W. Potter and Ron Warren, 'Humor as Camouflage of Televised Violence', *Journal of Communication* 48, no. 2

(1998): 40–57, https://doi.org/10.1111/j.1460-2466.1998.tb02747.x.

263 Ibid.

264 Ibid.

265 Eve M. Valera and Howard Berenbaum, 'Brain Injury in Battered Women', J *Consult Clin Psychol* 71, no. 4 (August 2003): 797–804, doi: 10.1037/0022-006x.71.4.797. PMID: 12924684.

266 Dr Eve M. Valera, interview with Hana Walker-Brown.

267 Eve M. Valera and Aaron Kucyi, 'Brain Injury in Women Experiencing Intimate Partner-Violence: Neural Mechanistic Evidence of an "Invisible" Trauma', *Brain Imaging Behav*. 11, no. 6 (December 2017): 1664–1677, doi: 10.1007/s11682-016-9643-1. PMID: 27766587.

268 Ibid.

269 Dr Eve M. Valera, interview with Hana Walker-Brown.

270 Ibid.

271 Ibid.

272 Judge Gibbs, *Gifts from the Ashes* (US: Xulon Press, 2017).

273 Dr Eve M. Valera, interview with Hana Walker-Brown.

274 'The Disabilities Trust Launches New Report: Making the Link: Female Offending and Brain Injury', *The United Kingdom Acquired Brain Injury Forum*, 12 February 2019, https://ukabif.org.uk/news/437830/The-Disabilities-Trust-Launches-New-Report-Making-the-Link-Female-Offending-and-Brain-Injury.htm.

275 'The Disabilities Trust Launch "Making the Link" Report', News, *The Disabilities Trust*, https://www.thedtgroup.org/foundation/news/the-disabilities-trust-launch-making-the-link-report.

276 *Ibid*.

277 'Female Offender Strategy', Ministry of Justice, Uk Parliament (June 2018), https://assets.publishing.service.gov.uk/government/uploads/system/uploads/attachment_data/file/719819/female-offender-strategy.pdf.

278 Ibid.

279 Lisa Marie Montgomery v Warden of USP Terre Haute, IN, et al., 'Order Granting Motion to Stay Execution Pending a Competence Hearing', United States District Court, 1 January 2021, https://drive.google.com/file/d/12M0YUcpt1FGUfy-c0aWfT-4NBkPnSEEht/view.

280 Bhargav Acharya and Robert Birsel, 'US Judge Blocks Execution of Only Woman on Federal Death Row', *Reuters*, 12 January 2021, https://www.reuters.com/world/us/us-judge-blocks-execution-only-woman-federal-death-row-2021-01-12/.

281 Tarig Tahir, Megan Palin and Mollie Mansfield, 'Lisa Montgomery "Throbbed" during Execution and "Licked Her Lips" as Lethal Injection Pumped through Body', *The US Sun*, last modified 14 January 2021, https://www.the-sun.com/news/2129539/lisa-montgomery-execution-bobbie-jo-stinnett-prayer/.

282 Laura Gesualdi-Gilmore, '"Womb Raider" Lisa Montgomery's Execution Blocked Hours before Her Lethal Injection in Dramatic 11th Hour Court Ruling', *The US Sun*, last modified 12 January 2021, https://www.the-sun.com/news/2122466/womb-raider-lisa-montgomery-woman-executed-70-years/.

283 Stephen T. Casper and Kelly O'Donnell, 'The Punch-Drunk Boxer and the Battered Wife: Gender and Brain Injury Research', *Social Science & Medicine* 245 (January 2020), https://doi.org/10.1016/j.socscimed.2019.112688.

284 Ibid.

285 Richard Schneider and Elizabeth Crosby, 'Physical Basis for Aggressive Assaultive Behavior in Football Players', in *Head and Neck Injuries in Football: Mechanisms, Treatment and Prevention*, ed. Richard Schneider (Baltimore: Williams and Wilkin's Co, 1973), p. 140.

286 '"Concussion" Doctor: "I Would Bet My Medical License" O.J. Simpson Has Degenerative Brain Disease CTE', *ABC News*, 29 January 2016, https://abcnews.go.com/US/concus-

sion-doctor-bet-medical-license-oj-simpson-degenerative/
story?id=36587331.

287   A *Times* staff writer, 'O.J. Simpson Chase: Cheering Fans, Curious Residents Joined Action', *Los Angeles Times*, 18 June 2014,
https://www.latimes.com/local/lanow/la-me-ln-oj-simp-
son-chase-cheering-fans-curious-residents-joined-action-
20140617-story.html.

288   Kirk Johnson, 'Prosecutors Drop Kobe Bryant Rape Case',
The New York Times, 2 September 2004, https://www.
nytimes.com/2004/09/02/us/prosecutors-drop-kobe-bry-
ant-rape-case.html.

289   'Kobe Bryant's Apology', *ESPN*, 2 September 2004, https://
www.espn.co.uk/nba/news/story?id=1872928.

290   Laura Collins, '"First Degree Rape… Lmao": Revealed,
Shocking Tweets at the Center of a Second Steubenville Rape
Claim', *The Daily Mail Online*, last modified 6 December
2013, https://www.dailymail.co.uk/news/article-2519570/
EXCLUSIVE-First-degree-rape--lmao--Shocking-tweets-
center-allegations-SECOND-Steubenville-rape-months-as-
sault-scandalised-America.html.

291   Don Carpenter, 'Leaked Steubenville Big Red Rape Video',
YouTube video, 2 January 2013, https://www.youtube.com/
watch?v=W1oahqCzwcY.

292   Nancy Schwartzman, *Roll Red Roll* (Chicago, United States:
Together Films, 2018).

293   https://www.latimes.com/nation/la-xpm-2013-mar-17-la-
na-nn-steubenville-mother-speaks-20130317-story.html.

294   https://www.reuters.com/article/us-usa-crime-ohio-idUS-
BRE9040BP20130105.

295   https://bigstory.ap.org/article/ohio-ag-plans-announcement-
about-rape-case-inquiry.

296   https://www.heraldstaronline.com/sports/local-
sports/2020/07/coach-reno-saccoccia-were-planning-to-
play-football-in-the-fall/.

297 https://www.motherjones.com/politics/2013/06/kyanony-mous-fbi-steubenville-raid-anonymous/.

298 https://www.justice.gov/usao-edky/pr/winches-ter-man-sentenced-24-months-illegally-hacking-web-site-and-lying-federal-agents.

299 Ibid.

300 http://prinniefied.com/wp/2012/12/27/case-dismissed/.

301 'California Judge Recalled for Sentence in Sexual Assault Case', Feminist Legal Theory, *Harvard Law Review*, 8 February 2019, https://harvardlawreview.org/2019/02/califor-nia-judge-recalled-for-sentence-in-sexual-assault-case/.

302 Katie J.M. Baker, 'Here's the Powerful Letter the Stanford Victim Read To Her Attacker', *Buzzfeed News*, 3 June 2016, https://www.buzzfeednews.com/article/katiejmbaker/heres-the-powerful-let-ter-the-stanford-victim-read-to-her-ra#.vcqERNAgKX.

303 Ibid.

304 Laith Al-Khalaf and Alexandra Topping, 'Over Half of UK Women Killed by Men Die at Hands of Partner or Ex', *The Guardian*, 20 February 2020, https://www.theguardian.com/uk-news/2020/feb/20/over-half-of-uk-women-killed-by-men-die-hands-current-ex-partner.

305 Dr Eve M. Valera, interview with Hana Walker-Brown.

306 Louis Theroux, 'FKA Twigs', *Grounded with Louise Theroux*, epi-sode 19, produced by Paul Kobrak, released 25 January 2021, https://www.bbc.co.uk/sounds/play/p091pg54.

307 Katherine Snedaker, interview with Hana Walker-Brown.

308 PINK Concussions, 'Cindy Parlow Cone at the NIH – PINK Panel', YouTube Video, posted 8 March 2018, https://www.youtube.com/watch?v=48_ciqoEMeM.

309 Ibid.

310 'PINK 1', *Pink Concussions*, https://www.pinkconcussions.com/pink-1.

311 Andrew E. Lincoln et al., 'Trends in Concussion Inci-dence in High School Sports: A Prospective 11-Year Study',

Am J Sports Med. 30, no. 5 (May 2011): 958–963, doi: 10.1177/0363546510392326.

Chapter Nine

312 Professor Adam J. White, interview with Hana Walker-Brown.

313 James Glenday, 'Should Tackling in School Rugby Be Banned?', *ABC Australia,* 3 March 2016, https://www.abc.net.au/am/content/2016/s4417627.htm.

314 Adam J. White et al., 'Open Letter: Removal of the Tackle in School Rugby', letter to Chief Medical Officers, 18 December 2020, https://allysonpollock.com/wp-content/uploads/2020/12/OpenLetterCMOs_2020-12-18.pdf.

315 Stephen A. Griffin et al., 'The Relationships between Rugby Union, and Health and Well-Being: A Scoping Review', *British Journal of Sports Medicine* 55 (March 2021): 319–326.

316 Robert Cantu, *Concussion and Our Kids: America's Leading Expert on How to Protect Young Athletes and Keep Sports Safe* (Boston: Mariner Books, 2013).

317 Rick Westhead, 'NHL in Legal Battle with Insurers Refusing to Pay Concussion Lawsuit Costs', *TSN,* 23 November 2020, https://www.tsn.ca/westhead-nhl-in-legal-battle-with-insurers-refusing-to-pay-concussion-lawsuit-costs-1.1555455.

318 Dr Robert Cantu, interview with Hana Walker-Brown.

319 Ibid.

320 Mark Fainaru-Wada and Steve Fainaru, 'NFL Backs Away from Funding BU Brain Study; NIH to Fund It Instead', *ESPN,* 21 December 2015, https://www.espn.com/espn/otl/story/_/id/14417386/nfl-pulls-funding-boston-university-head-trauma-study-concerns-researcher.

321 Ibid.

322 'Almost Half of Sport Injury-Related A&E Attendances Are Children', Press Office, Newcastle University, 2 November 2018, https://www.ncl.ac.uk/press/articles/archive/2018/11/sportinjury/.

323 Allyson Pollock, *Tackling Rugby: What Every Parent Should Know* (London: Verso Books, 2014).

324 'Sports Injury Statistics', *Stanford Children's Health*, https://www.stanfordchildrens.org/en/topic/default?id=sports-injury-statistics-90-P02787.

325 'Sports Injury Statistics', *Stanford Children's Health*.

326 Dr Bennett Omalu, interview with Hana Walker-Brown.

327 'Routine Hits Playing Football Cause Damage to the Brain', *Science Daily*, 7 August 2019, https://www.sciencedaily.com/releases/2019/08/190807142249.htm.

328 Ibid.

329 Ibid.

330 Reid Forgrave, 'The Concussion Diaries: One High School Football Player's Secret Struggle with CTE', Culture, GQ, 10 January 10, 2017, https://www.gq.com/story/the-concussion-diaries-high-school-football-cte

331 Bill Littlefield, '"He Knew Football Had Everything to Do With It": A CTE Journal', Only a. Game, *WBUR*, 2 February 2018, https://www.wbur.org/onlyagame/2018/02/02/zac-easter-cte-concussion-football.

332 John Gaal Sr, interview with Hana Walker-Brown.

333 Peter Robinson, Twitter, https://twitter.com/peterrobinson86/media.

334 John Gaal Sr, interview with Hana Walker-Brown.

Chapter Ten

335 Andy Bull, '"They Are Going to Come After You": A Doctor's Advice on Rugby's Battle over Brain Injury', Sport, *The Guardian*, 29 March 2021, https://www.theguardian.com/sport/2021/mar/29/they-are-going-to-come-after-you-a-doctors-advice-on-rugbys-battle-over-brain-injuries.

336 Sam Peters, interview with Hana Walker-Brown.

337 Ibid.

338 https://www.dailymail.co.uk/sport/concussion/index.html.

339 Ibid.

340 Steve Thompson, interview with Hana Walker-Brown.
341 Ibid.
342 'Alix Popham: Ex-Wales flanker on Early Onset Dementia Diagnosis', Rugby Union, *BBC*, 8 December 2020, https://www.bbc.co.uk/sport/rugby-union/55208227.
343 Ibid.
344 Bull, '"They Are Going to Come After You"'.
345 Ibid.
346 'Rugby and Brain Injuries: Way Players Train Should Be Addressed "Very Quickly"', Rugby Union, *BBC*, 10 December 2020, https://www.bbc.co.uk/sport/rugby-union/55253926.
347 'Update 1-Rugby-Endland World Cup Winner Thompson Reveals Dementia Diagnosis,' *Reuters*, 8 December 2020, https://www.reuters.com/article/rugby-union-concussion-idINL1N2IO2D6.
348 'Concussion in Rugby: Is Rugby Safe for Kids?', News Round, *BBC*, 30 September 2021, https://www.bbc.co.uk/newsround/57795018.
349 Eanna Falvey, 'How World Rugby's Concussion Return to Play Protocol Works', *World Rugby*, 3 February 2021, https://www.world.rugby/news/613856/how-world-rugbys-concussion-return-to-play-protocol-works.
350 'An Open Letter to Sir Bill Beaumont, Chairman of World Rugby', *Progressive Rugby*, https://www.progressiverugby.com/open-letter.
351 'World Rugby Statement in Response to Progressive Rugby Group Player Welfare Proposals', *World Rugby*, 18 February 2021, https://www.world.rugby/news/617530/declaration-world-rugby-reponse-propositions-amelioration-sante-joueurs.
352 Judith Gates, interview with Hana Walker-Brown.
353 Ibid.
354 Ibid.
355 'Who We Are,' *Head for Change*, https://headforchange.org.uk/who-we-are/.

356 Stephen T. Casper et al., 'Toward Complete, Candid, and Unbiased International Consensus Statements on Concussion in Sport', *Journal of Law, Medicine & Ethics* 49, no. 3 (2021): 372–377, doi:10.1017/jme.2021.56.

357 David Kriebel et al., 'The Precautionary Principle in Environmental Science', *Environmental Health Perspectives* 109, no. 9 (2001): 871–876, doi: 10.1289/ehp.01109871.

358 Ibid.

359 Jem Aswad, 'The Weeknd Reveals the Significance of His Full-Face Bandages, Ahead of SuperBowl (EXCLUSIVE)', *Variety*, 3 February 2021, https://variety.com/2021/music/news/the-weeknd-bandages-super-bowl-plastic-surgery-1234898743.

360 'Concussion in Sport', Committees, UK Parliament, https://committees.parliament.uk/work/977/concussion-in-sport/news/.

361 'DCMS Committee to Consider Links between Sport and Long-Term Brain Injury', Committees, UK Parliament, 3 March 2021, https://committees.parliament.uk/work/977/concussion-in-sport/news/146543/dcms-committee-to-consider-links-between-sport-and-longterm-brain-injury/.

362 'Tuesday 27 April Meeting', Digital, Culture, Media and Sport (DCMS) Committee, Parliament Live TV, 27 April 2021, https://www.parliamentlive.tv/Event/Index/3e7a8b14-8287-4221-a278-a87d3e995aeb.

363 Ibid.

364 'Tuesday 9 March 2021 Meeting', Digital, Culture, Media and Sport (DCMS) Committee, Parliament Live TV, 9 March 2021, https://parliamentlive.tv/event/index/d78a3d5f-2036-4667-9929-57d7b216746f?in=10:00:07.

365 'Concussion in Sport: Third Report of Session 2021-22', *House of Commons*, 15 July 2021, https://committees.parliament.uk/publications/6879/documents/72591/default/.

366 'Concussion in Sport Inquiry', News, The PFA, 22 July 2021, https://www.thepfa.com/news/2021/7/22/the-pfa-concussion-in-sport-inquiry.

367 'Heading in Football: Professional Players in England Limited to 10 "Higher Force Headers" a Week in Training', Sport, *BBC*, 28 July 2021, https://www.bbc.co.uk/sport/football/57996593.

368 Emma R. Russel, 'Association of Field Position and Career Length with Risk of Neurodegenerative Disease in Male Former Professional Soccer Players', *JAMA Neurol.* 78, no. 9 (September 2021): 1057–1063, http://eprints.gla.ac.uk/248747/.

369 Jeremy Wilson, 'Football's dementia crisis research shows just 20 "normal" headers can lead to concussion test failure,' *The Telegraph,* November 17, 2020, https://www.telegraph.co.uk/football/2020/11/17/footballs-dementia-crisis-research-shows-just-20-normal-headers/

370 '"Totally Ridiculous": Fans Unimpressed at "Do-Gooders" Urging Football Bosses to Ask "Difficult Questions" about Outlawing Headers', *RT International*, 3 August 2021, https://www.rt.com/sport/531010-dementia-football-heading-ball-research/.

371 Statement to Author.

372 Sir Bill Beaumont, 'An Open Letter by Sir Bill Beaumont: Striving to Be the Most Progressive Sport for Player Welfare', News, *World Rugby*, 13 July 2021, https://www.world.rugby/news/653081.

373 'Head Impact Prevention & Management Plan Announced for Professional Game,' News, *England Rugby*, 22 July 2021, https://www.englandrugby.com/news/article/head-impact-prevention-management-plan-announced-for-professional-game.

374 'The Drake Foundation Urges Review into Laws of Professional Era Rugby Union as Study Suggests Sport May Have Been Safer in the Amateur Era', Latest News, *The Drake Foundation*, 20 October 2021, https://www.drakefoundation.org/the-drake-foundation-urges-review-into-laws-of-professional-era-rugby-union-as-study-suggests-sport-may-have-been-safer-in-the-amateur-ersa/.

375 'The PFA Call for Industry-Wide Care Fund', *The PFA*, 28 October 2021, https://www.thepfa.com/news/2021/10/28/pfa-call-for-industry-wide-care-fund.

376 Melissa Davey, Stephanie Convery and Emma Kemp, 'New plagiarism claims against sport concussion guru Paul McCrory', *The Guardian*, 22 September 2022, https://www.theguardian.com/sport/2022/sep/23/new-plagiarism-claims-against-sport-concussion-guru-paul-mccrory.

377 AFL, 'Independent Review – Associate Professor Paul McCrory', 25 October 2022, https://www.afl.com.au/news/860719/independent-review-associate-professor-paul-mccrory.

378 Angus Fontaine, 'Concussion kingpin resigns from global post over plagiarism scandal', *The Guardian*, 5 March 2022, https://www.theguardian.com/sport/2022/mar/05/concussion-kingpin-resigns-global-post-over-plagiarism-scandal.

379 BJSM, 'Retraction: The time lords – measurement and performance in sprinting', 3 October 2022, https://bjsm.bmj.com/content/early/2022/10/06/bjsports-39-11-785ret.

380 BMJ, 'British Journal of Sports Medicine retracts further 9 articles authored by former editor in chief', EurekAlert!, 10 October 2022, https://www.eurekalert.org/news-releases/967118; Helen Macdonald et al., 'Update on the investigation into the publication record of former BJSM editor-in-chief Paul McCrory', *British Journal of Sports Medicine*, 17 November 2022, https://bjsm.bmj.com/content/early/2022/10/07/bjsports-2022-106408.

381 Christopher J. Nowinski et al., 'Applying the Bradford Hill Criteria for Causation to Repetitive Head Impacts and Chronic Traumatic Encephalopathy', *Frontiers in Neurology*, 22 July 2022, https://doi.org/10.3389/fneur.2022.938163.

382 Barry Wilner, 'NFL awarding more than $35 million to brain injury studies', *The Durango Herald*, 16 November 2018, https://www.durangoherald.com/articles/nfl-awarding-more-than-35-million-to-brain-injury-studies/.

383 Ken Belson, 'Scientists Say Concussions Can Cause a Brain Disease. These Doctors Disagree', *New York Times*, 8 November 2022, https://www.nytimes.com/2022/11/08/sports/football/cte-brain-trauma-concussions.html.